The Flower Healer

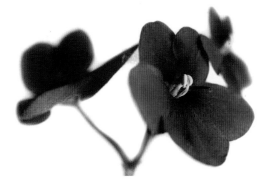

The Flower Healer

Flower-essence medicine for healing

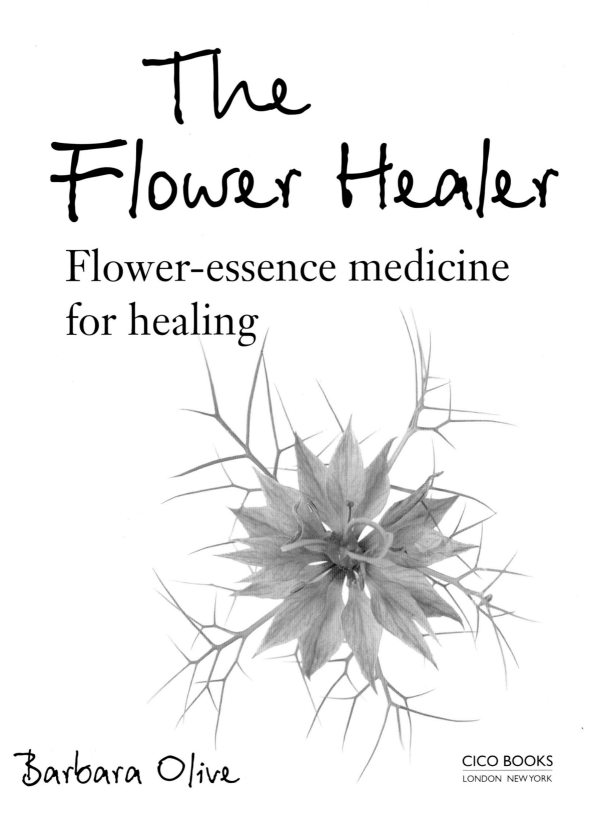

Barbara Olive

CICO BOOKS
LONDON NEW YORK

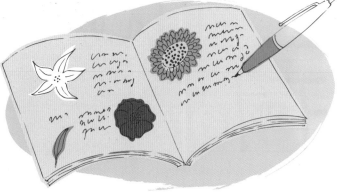

First published in 2007 by CICO Books
an imprint of Ryland Peters & Small
20–21 Jockey's Fields, London WC1R 4BW

10 9 8 7 6 5 4 3 2 1

Text © Barbara Olive 2007
Design and illustrations © CICO Books 2007
Cover photograph: Tony Howell/Flowerphotos.
For photography credits, see page 144.

A CIP catalogue record for this book is available from the British Library

ISBN-13: 978 1 904991 60 1
ISBN-10: 1 904991 60 2

Editor: Marie Clayton
Designer: David Fordham
Picture research: Robin Gurdon
Illustrations: Trina Dalziel

Printed in China

NOTE

The plants described in this book, when used as flower or vibrational essences, do not have the same effect
on the body as herbal and chemical compounds or essential oils. It you are taking any other preparation
made from a derivative of these plants, taking the corresponding flower or vibrational essence at the same
time will not do any harm and will help to ease the emotional cause of the problem.

Contents

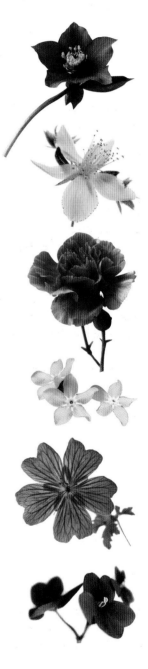

A Healing Path

Above:
The lovely Stargazer Lily soothes the emotions holding back creativity and allows energy to flow freely, increasing feelings of self-worth, love and positivity.

My own journey with complementary medicine started 15 years ago, when my eldest son was diagnosed with Attention Deficit Disorder at the age of two. At the time, it was hard for me to look at anything other than conventional medicine – after all, I'd been a nurse almost all my working life. Although I felt guilty about the idea of seeking help via a less conventional route, my gut instinct told me that I needed to start looking elsewhere – and I have spent my entire life being guided by my thoughts and instincts.

I had learned at a very early age to trust the messages from my spirit guides. I always knew that there was something different about their voices – that they were not simply my imagination – and I learned to trust them more than I could trust any human being. These were the voices that told me to run away from danger, and when I didn't listen, I got hurt. So, being an intuitive and clairvoyant from birth, I was happy to be guided by my inner tuition and my spirit helpers and to find the assistance my son required wherever I could.

I looked at all the alternative therapies, including homoeopathy and acupuncture, weighed up the positives and negatives of each therapy and finally started using essences, first on my son and then on myself. With flower essences, unlike other remedies, I was encouraged by the fact that if I gave him the wrong essence there would be no effect at all and if I did manage to find the correct one the only side effect would be an emotional one – for the better. Gradually he began to get better – and so did I.

With this positive experience under my belt, I began my own amazing journey. I was then working as a spiritual counsellor and medium and at the conclusion of a session my client would be advised by spirit to look at supplements, vitamins, yoga, physical exercise and then Bach Flower Remedies. I would ask spirit why the client needed Crab Apple, for instance, and they would answer. I made copious notes and day-by-day I learned about the fascinating world of Dr Bach and his insight into flowers and their abilities to heal. Soon I joined forces with a flower essence therapist, who would administer the essences after confirming they were appropriate. As if by magic, everything seemed to work harmoniously for everyone. I was also taking classes in Bach Flower Therapy and soon my teacher suggested I make them myself for clients, so I promptly picked up the phone to order a practitioner set of Bach Flowers. A few days later a complete set of Bush Flower Essences arrived at my door – how on earth did that happen? Coincidence? For me, this wrong delivery meant that I needed to start learning about more flower essences, and so the lessons from spirit continued.

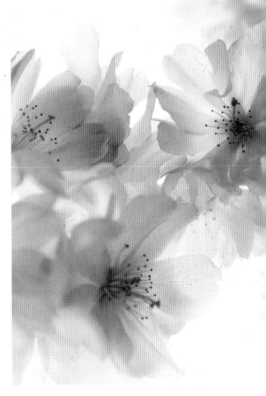

Next I took classes with Ian White, founder of Australian Bush Flower Essences. My guidance was being confirmed; everything they had told me was being validated time and time again. I made my first essence during this mad period of learning and loved the experience. It took me a full day and I was totally immersed in the whole process. When my first essence, Blackberry, was complete I started to take it, and I quickly found that it was helping me to address many issues that I had been dealing with – such as the identity challenges I was struggling to come to terms with, letting go of my old life, feeling very alone in my pursuits and having no control over what was happening in my personal life. I felt that I was moving forward in leaps and bounds. At this time I was spending 15 minutes or so every day out in the park, and I would communicate with the trees – this first began when I walked past a Snow Gum tree and instantly felt such a profound sense of connection. The following day a flyer arrived in the post for a course on Sabian Tree Essences with Judi Harvey, their founder – this was synchronicity at its best. Another 18 months of studying, and my understanding of the medicine became deeper and deeper.

A sudden move to England in 1998 forced me to leave my practice and my beloved trees behind. Feeling very homesick for Australia, I started teaching the Tree Essence practitioner course myself and felt instantly back in touch with 'my friends'. Then I was invited to the inaugural meeting of the British Flower and Vibrational Essence Association (BFVEA) and a whole new world opened before me. I was like a child in a sweet shop – I wanted everything and I had so many new

Above:
Flower petals are direct communication from nature, encouraging us to touch, stroke and smell a flower to link directly with its energy.

friends who shared the same interests. Every plant, flower and tree had new meaning and the world around me, once only a picture, became alive. A trip to Norway brought an intoxicating influx of even more sensations, as I was now learning about water, ice and its effects and possibilities within the essence repertoire. Was there any end to this? It seemed the more I learned, the more I realized what I didn't know.

The questions from within came thick and fast. I had come so far from the world of conventional medicine that I had loved so much, surely there must be a connection – worlds could not live side by side like this without overlapping. I 'knew' the world needed to experience this other side. Mark Wells, an author and lecturer on Bach Essences from Melbourne, refers to this as 'knowing with a "K", or knowing with a "G" ' (a reference to the Greek word *gnosis* which literally means knowledge). So what did I do? I started Essence World, supplying essences to anyone who wanted them. Months later, the website was up, the shop and clinic in Eton opened … and then I asked the fateful question to my ever-present teachers, 'Come on, guys, now tell me how essences really work.' Their answer was immediate: 'You're asking how to tie a shoelace, and you don't even know what the shoe looks like.' The only way to interpret what they were saying was to acknowledge that I had no idea of the structure of energy. So, from that day, I began another teaching session that continues to this day. My somewhat simple beliefs about energy were crumpled and discarded – my guides were showing me something I'd never read nor studied before. I was learning *exactly* where and how essences worked, the tiny strands, the huge fuse boxes and multipart valves that are the framework of our intricate energy system.

I am so in awe of this that I don't have the words to describe my thirst for the truth or my appreciation of all my teachers, physical and in spirit. I still feel astonishment how, every time I give an essence, energy shifts in my patients – and how quickly they then develop and find happiness and contentment, sometimes for the first time in their lives. I want everyone to be able to experience the power of essences, and to teach those who don't have the power of clear second sight to find ways of using their intuition so they are able to work with essences easily.

Please join me in opening a new world for you.

Opposite:
Pincushion, or Leucospermum, helps increase your force field so you may touch the lives of others in a positive way and encourage them to follow your lead.

CAUTION: If you have a serious mental or emotional condition, or a known physical medical problem, you should seek the care or advice of a qualified health practitioner. Flower essences are not a cure for such serious conditions – however, their use may help to halt the problem and, more importantly, help you to understand why you have these symptoms and ailments in order to allow healing to take place. Many health practitioners now include flower essences in their health programmes, or work with other practitioners who do.

I want everyone to be
able to experience
the power of
flower essences

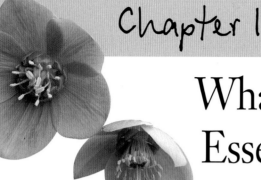

Chapter 1

What are Flower Essences?

Above:
Hellebore flower
essence helps you to
accept change.

The healing powers of flowers have been lovingly used for centuries, across the world and throughout civilization. The ancient Greeks and Egyptians held Nature itself as a religious symbol, and flowers, plants and trees were deemed to be a gift from the gods and to hold many powers of virtue, luck, love and divine protection from evil. Temples and sacred places were often built in areas of outstanding natural beauty, and flowers were believed to have spiritual and supernatural powers. The Egyptians surrounded their deceased loved ones with flowers to ensure a safe journey into the next life and even today we bring flowers to the graveside and to brighten the spirits of a sick friend.

Flower essences are energy or vibrational infusions, made from the spirit of a plant by floating the plant in a crystal bowl of spring water, usually under sunlight. The first 38 flower remedies were formulated in the 1930s by the renowned British physician Dr Edward Bach, who discovered a method of imbuing pure water with the healing properties of herbs and wildflowers. He went on to create the Bach Flower Remedies, which are still used and universally recognized.

Today there are an ever-increasing number of essences made from plants and living elements, including gemstones and even waterfalls. Indeed, the flower used on the cover of this book – South African Daisy (*Osteospermum jucundum*) – had never existed as an essence, until its image was chosen by the publishers as a symbol of the book. 'But it's not an essence,' I told them. 'But we love this picture!' they replied. 'But it's not an essence!!' I continued, bemused at their obstinacy. Then I thought to myself... perhaps, just perhaps, this is another flower just begging to be immortalized in an essence and maybe this is the energy of *The Flower Healer*.

My first task was to find the correct species. There are at least 50 different Osteospermums to choose from, but no less than 10 minutes later – with the help of the Internet – I had the name. Now I had to find out where I could get hold of one that had been nurtured and cared for as much as any nursery or garden centre could. Never having purchased a plant before with the express notion of making an essence, this was a new experience for me. The Beth Chatto Gardens, on the outskirts of Colchester in Essex, were an inspiration. My only regret was that I didn't have time to explore further than my purchase – I was on my way to The Bach Cromer Conference and a celebration of the life of Dr Bach who, had he still been alive, would have been 120 years old. It seemed that synchronicity was hard at work here; even the Osteospermums went to the conference!

Researching the plant, I found out that it's also known as *Osteospermum barberae* and a shiver reverberated throughout my body – no, this is just too much. What are the chances of Barbara's book flower also being called Barbara? My publishers must be geniuses. My South African Daisy, or SAD for short, was beginning to take on a life of its own. Back in Berkshire I captured a window of sunshine that had been eluding us for weeks and my plants produced four beautiful flowers to be used for the essence. I talked to the plants every day encouraging them to flower, although it was now October and not the best time to make any essence, since sunshine – and lots of it – is an extremely important ingredient. Essences can also be made under the influence of the moon, but this flower closes its petals as soon as the sun and light start to fade, and both it and I wanted the blooms to be open to the world to show what a beautiful being it could truly be.

Below:
Essences can be made either under the influence of sunlight or by moonlight, but ideally the blooms should be wide open to the world.

Creating a New Essence

Osteosperma/Osteospermum comes from the Greek *osteon*, meaning 'bone' and *sperma*, which used as part of a compound word in Greek means '-seeded' – thus the name means 'hard-seeded'. Ostoespermum is closely related to the small genus Chrysanthemoide. It has a very faint smell of the Chrysanthemum and the daisy-like flowers are a lovely silvery pink with a yellow eye, which becomes blue in the centre as it matures. Each day the blue grows and the yellow diminishes, until it finally fades to a yellow rim around a blue eye. I'm addicted to it. So let's look at some of its attributes or its personality. This wants to be on the cover of the book, not inside, so it's really ambitious. Its name equates to hard-seed. So let's say it's quite hard to grow and, through a profound process, will eventually open up and shine. It says, 'I'm going for it.'

So once it has found its voice, with maturity and experience, it can stand on its own. Now this is spooky – it really does sound like me. It's a well-known fact we make essences for ourselves first and foremost, and I was now beginning to believe it. With very little time to prove the essence and give you some vital information, I employed the help of Alison McCabe, a South African colleague, who compiles the most amazing birth charts and information on your personality relating to the time of your birth. I gave her the time and place of Osty's birth – I can't call it SAD any more, because it is so far from sad.

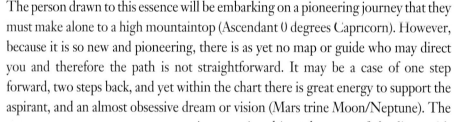

Birth Chart for the 'South African Daisy' Person

The South African Daisy was born as an essence on October 3rd, 2006, in my garden at Sunninghill, Berkshire, England.

Below:
The South African Daisy, which did not exist as an essence until its image was chosen by the publishers of this book.

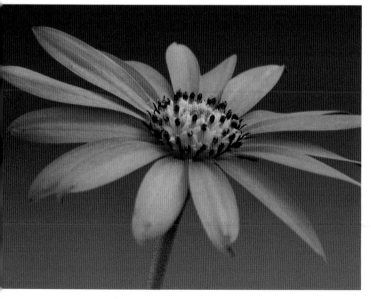

The person drawn to this essence will be embarking on a pioneering journey that they must make alone to a high mountaintop (Ascendant 0 degrees Capricorn). However, because it is so new and pioneering, there is as yet no map or guide who may direct you and therefore the path is not straightforward. It may be a case of one step forward, two steps back, and yet within the chart there is great energy to support the aspirant, and an almost obsessive dream or vision (Mars trine Moon/Neptune). The journey is ultimately one of healing with Chiron, the wounded healer in the first house. The path up this mountain is a hard one. It brings to mind the pioneers who first crossed southern Africa in horse-drawn wagons through treacherous mountains and deserts to find a place they could call home.

There is much in the chart to suggest that although there is a powerful vision (Neptune/ Moon conjunct in the first house) there is also the quality of a 'mirage' that comes with this placement of Neptune, such that the person may sometimes doubt the way ahead. There are also other forces that constantly frustrate the person on their journey (Saturn opposing

Neptune/Moon and Jupiter squaring Saturn and Neptune/Moon). There is an almost constant struggle and tension between what the person perceives in their visionary ideal and the realities of the constraints of everyday life. Pluto, god of deep transformation, is also perfectly square to the Moon's north node, indicating that the destiny of the chart is frustrated. The north node of the chart is in Pisces – that again brings in the idealism and vision of beauty that urge the person on in their quest. It is in the second house ruled by Mercury, god of communication.

The Sun in the chart is in Libra in the ninth house of long distance travel and higher education. This brings a quality of balance; the person's vision is supported by their higher education and their many life experiences, giving it substance. Mars and Venus lie to either side of the Sun bringing a sense of harmony of male and female forces within the essence. This trio in the chart is also reflected in the colours of the flower – pink petals (Venus), yellow centre (Sun) and blue core centre (Mars).

This journey may twist and turn, often leaving the person feeling pulled in many directions at once, but they will almost certainly not give up. This person has a truly pioneering spirit (Sun quincunx Uranus) and will always find creative ways to overcome any barrier put before them. They will also be incredibly tough, as were the earliest pioneers. The chart also has a strong 'Mars quality' bringing immense will and energy to the person.

The highest outcome of the 'African Daisy' person is communication from a place of deep experience and transformation. Having being thrown into the flames of alchemy, and shown unrelenting will to succeed, the person emerges renewed with great strength and purpose (Mercury conjunct the mid heaven in Scorpio). The element of 'beauty' is also strongly suggested here.

The Latin name of the plant translates to 'hard seed'. This aspect of the plant's personality is very much evident in the birth chart of the essence. This is truly an alchemical journey that results in the growth of a flower of most stunning beauty and grace. The South African Daisy essence is a cup of sweet nectar for a person whose life is full of transformation and striving for their ideals. It can strengthen the positive aspects of will, balance and vision, whilst bringing acceptance of the hardships along the way as part of the experience that ultimately brings a startling beauty.

Vibrational Energy

To truly understand how flower essences work requires an acceptance that we are more than just a physical body, that we also incorporate a 'body' of life energy – a life force – a 'body' of sensitivity and feelings and a spiritual essence. Flower essences are the energetic imprints of the life force of plants, which interact with these subtle bodies of ours and have an effect upon us. You might say they work in a similar way to inspirational music or art, which carries meaning – a vibration – through the medium of sound or light. Flower essences simply work through the medium of water. So consider for one moment – is not our body approximately 73 percent water (just like the earth itself)? We are a river, a tidal wave of vibrational energy ourselves, from the brain's cerebral fluid, the spinal fluid, lymphatic fluid in the tissues, synovial fluid in the joints – why, even the very amniotic fluid that held us before we came into this world. Energy all around us vibrates; we just have to find the right pitch, and the body, mind and emotion will work in harmony.

Above:
The common Thistle heals old wounds to the heart, helping to banish denial of intimacy and the fear of being unloved.

Energetically Speaking

In the known universe everything vibrates, from low frequency to high. Electrons, protons and neutrons, which form atoms and subatomic particles, all move at incredible speeds. All strains of science, quantum physics, religion, conventional medicine and complementary medicine have their own theories and rules by which their beliefs are proven, written and lived by. There are many arguments between rival factions throughout these groups, about who's right and who's wrong – the big bang theory versus evolution. What many of us have failed to realize is that by adding just one little factor, every single one of us is put into our rightful place in the plan or on the map. That one little factor is *energy*.

Energy is a product in its own right and has its own set of rules that it adheres to. Like electricity, it needs cabling, wires, terminals, fuses and a completed circuitry for it to be effective. Every living thing is infused by a universal energy that connects and nourishes all life. Over the centuries, often by Eastern civilizations more spiritual than our own, this energy has been called by many different names, such as 'subtle energy', 'prana', 'qi' and 'chi'. An 'invisible' energy field composed of this life force surrounds each human being. It is this energy field around and through each and every one of us that supports the life process in all

vibrational healing
can be used
to clear any
negative
thought forms

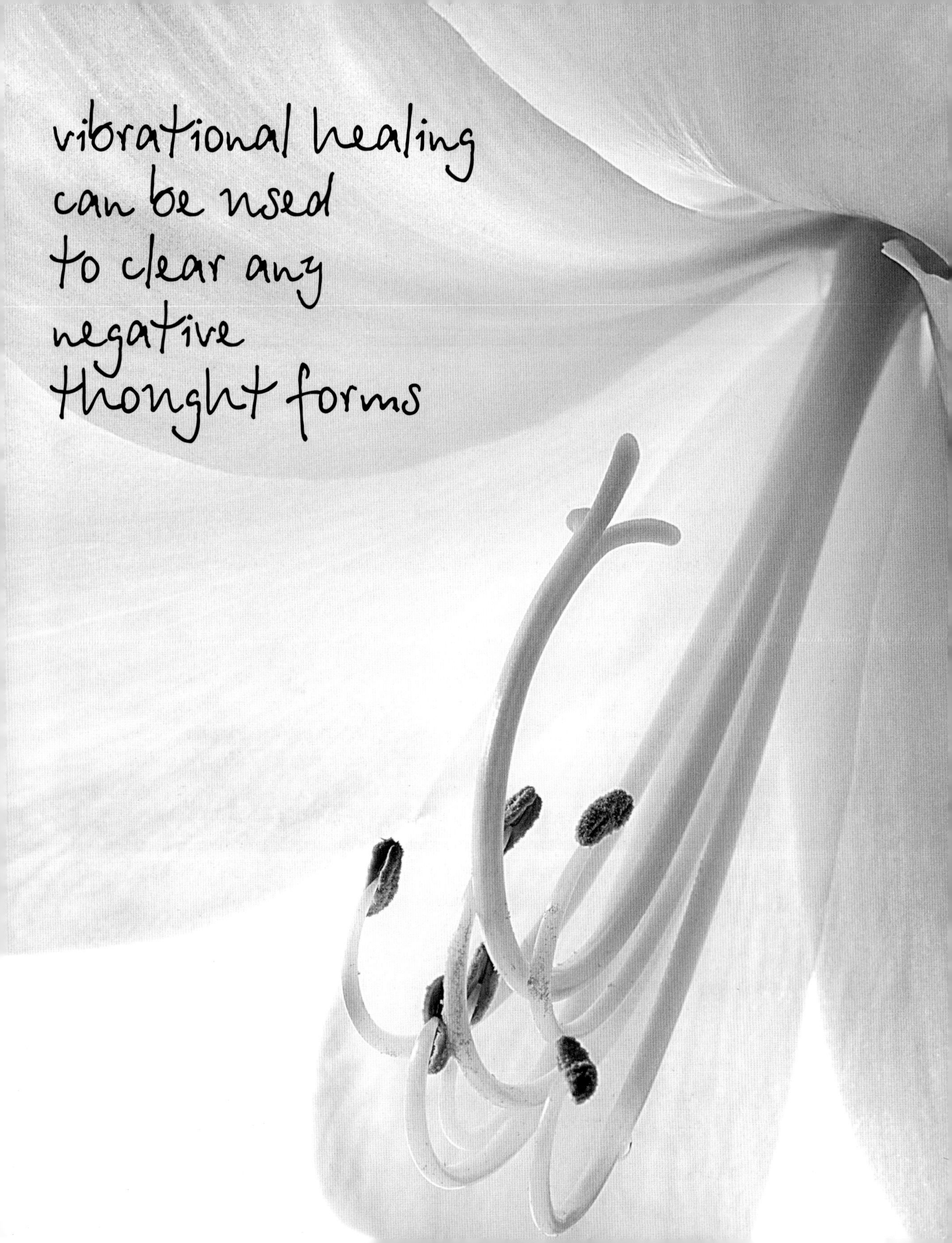

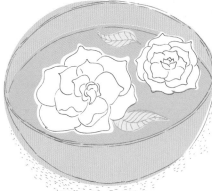

Flower essences are energy or vibrational infusions, made from the spirit of a plant by floating the plant in a crystal bowl of spring water – usually under sunlight.

its aspects – the physical body, the mind and our emotions, and the spiritual life. If you try to make sense of life by what you see as your own reality you can't – we are as different to one another as our fingerprints prove! But if you look at all the facts from an energy perspective, we are as one.

Just as we are not physically able to see subatomic particles, atoms, or molecules, neither do we experience the spirit world in the same way. We experience the world by using our heightened five senses, but beyond the five we have a sixth. The sixth sense is a combination of our awareness of the spiritual world, our intuition, and the psychic ability that we all have to some degree. Some simply tune into that vibrational frequency more easily than others. I guess that's me.

When everything is working in unison, we feel physically, emotionally and mentally healthy. When something is out of balance, then both our physical and energetic systems are functioning at less than maximum capacity. Physically, you may experience aches, pains, infections, loss of circulation/body function – and in more severe or out-of-balance cases, diseases, cancer and a host of illnesses caused by a lowered immune system. Mental and emotional imbalances might show as bipolar tendencies or anxiety, membrane imbalances as a martyr mentality, fear or anger, and spiritual imbalances as depression. These out-of-balance concerns may be as a result of countless reasons, including a physical accident, an emotional trauma, our body lacking the trace minerals, vitamins and nutrients it requires, not drinking enough water to hydrate the cells, and negative or toxic energies trapped in the various layers of our energy system. Each of the above will affect our energy system in some manner, through either an energy blockage or an imbalance, and our energy system affects our physical body. It's a complex, interconnected puzzle that, when seen as a whole, is both fascinating and sacred. The flow of energy goes to every part of our body, right down to the smallest cell, and radiates from within us to encapsulate our entire energy field. The energy communication centres in our physical body are known as chakras. Originating from Eastern philosophies, chakras – or energy/spiritual centres, as they're also known – are spinning wheels or vortexes that are responsible for the condition of our mind, body and spirit (see page 22).

Among other things, vibrational healing can be used to clear negative thought forms; rebalance and facilitate harmony within; increase vitality; and heal at the subtle level. Sometimes, for whatever reason, we hold onto negative thought forms. These thought patterns are created over a period of time, either by our own feelings and experiences – anger at someone, hatred, or because of a victim mentality, for example – or by allowing the impact someone has on us to take hold – the opposite of what would be called 'water off a duck's back'. When blockages build up in the energy centres due to internal and external stressors, we can feel pretty bad and low on energy. My boys have the ability to see energy as I do – when they were little, they would make negative thought forms from the energy in their bedroom by focusing negative thoughts on an object, just for something to do! They would then go into the garden to play and forget about them, so when they came back into their room they would get the fright of their life and run out, shouting that there were monsters in there. But, like any good mother should, I taught them to clean up their own mess and they soon realized it wasn't so much fun when mum left the room exactly as they had left it, so this game was soon over. Imagine those monsters inside you, though. Yuk!

How do I know this and why am I so convinced? I received proof one day five years ago. My marriage had been a struggle, to say the least. We had been married for 18 years, and during all of this time we had both lived our lives in our own realities. I had tried to love and be loved, but my thoughts constantly, every day, were, 'What have I done wrong?' I thought hard, right back to as far as I could remember, and I realized – having had a somewhat fractured childhood – that I had been asking this question my entire life. So I took an essence that I had made recently, Tears of Christ (for injustice and martyr mentality), and settled back to think some more. I seemed to have spent a lot of my childhood hiding from conflict; lying low meant that I stayed out of trouble, a coping technique I had employed from that moment on.

Below: *When a flower essence is made (see page 27) a snapshot of the energy of the flower is held in the water as a memory.*

I had tried everything possible to find a resolution for this behaviour, but I had always fallen into the same traps. I had seen counsellors, hypnotherapists, psychologists and every manner of alternative therapist; nothing they either said or suggested made any lasting difference to any of my problems, physical, emotional or mental. I ached physically, hurting deep in my bones and tendons, and I had experienced frozen shoulders for four years. It seemed that there was only one person who could do anything about this – me!

So what had I done? Mistake number one

was assuming that I had any control over someone else's reactions. You can only be responsible for your own actions. What other people do is their business, not yours. Blaming myself for over 40 years for other people's stuff had led to me having no self-esteem, no confidence, and very little care for myself – to the point that I was now becoming very ill physically. This was my journey, and the sooner I got that message, the happier I would be. I knew that the only thing stopping me was 'me', but how was I to change that? What did I need to do?

The answer was to stop blaming myself, to stop the negative self-talk. To not give away my energy to other people. I was getting the message and at that moment I decided to bring all my available energy back to myself from places I'd long forgotten about. We all have 100 percent energy available at any one time, but where was mine at that precise moment?

60 percent	Husband
35 percent	Children
5 percent	Household stuff

Below:
One way of taking your essence is to add the drops to a glass of pure spring water.

So there was none left for me. I decided there and then to bring all my energy back from everywhere, every single little bit. The realization of what I was doing was overwhelming – I imagined tentacles coming out of my body pumping the energy out of me so I just pulled all the tentacles back into myself. The force of this physically moved the chair I was sitting on and for the first time in my life I felt empowered. 'What have I done?' I asked again, but this time I knew what I had done and that I was 100 percent responsible. Still sitting in my study and looking around me, everything seemed more real, more solid. The trees and foliage looked brighter, my hearing was more acute. How much energy do we give away at any one time? I was about to find out: 'Barb,' said my husband, 'I've just had the weirdest feeling, as if I've just lost all my energy. I feel really ill.' I don't think I could answer – the confirmation of what I had just done was so profound that I didn't know what to say.

Giving away your energy to another is detrimental to you both. Don't get me wrong, this is fine as a short-term measure to help another over a particular situation – we all need a helping hand occasionally – but as a long-term prospect, without, it seems, your prior knowledge or consent, it is damaging. So how do you give away your energy unawares? Easily – by altering your actions to sustain another's apparent happiness, just like me as a child, and afterward when I spent my whole life trying to keep the peace for fear of reprisals.

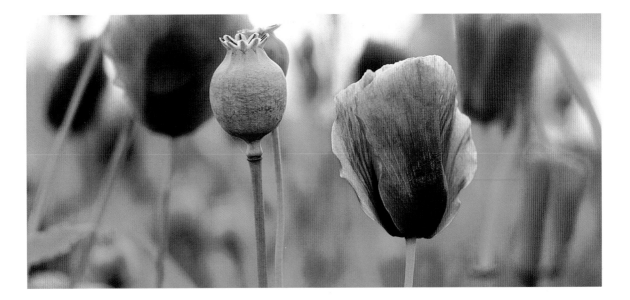

As there are 'givers', so there are 'energy stealers', or those who take. In his book *The Celestine Prophecy* (Bantam), James Redfield describes the energy stealer succinctly. Every one of us knows how to be one – use the 'poor me' look. Everyone around asks what is wrong, and you have an instant hook into them. Couples in some relationships give and take in these ways all the time; it is known as a codependent partnership. One needs to take, the other to give, so it would seem a perfect partnership – but it's not healthy. Both parties are living in altered realities and not being true to themselves; they are acting out plays because at some stage in their life they altered their energy flow to avoid being hurt.

Let's take this further, by looking at the past and how it can affect the circuits. Our physical body has a history: where it was made, the manufacturer, time and date of initial production, date of final completion of the product. Or, the date, time and place of conception, who your parents are, what defects their DNA carries and, more importantly, what energetic changes and foibles they have themselves that affect their personalities. And finally, the date, time and place of birth – the astrological implications. Your name can also affect this history: usually your parents choose your name and it reflects the merging of their personalities, with a little help from their intuition. The science of numerology can help you to understand your own unique fingerprint just by plotting the date of your birth and your name. This is a fascinating subject that I recommend you read more about in numerous excellent books, including my favourite, *The Life You Were Born to Live* by Dan Millman (H J Kramer). Just about everything you can think of has its

Above:
Flower essences have no side effects and their vibrational medicine can help everyone.

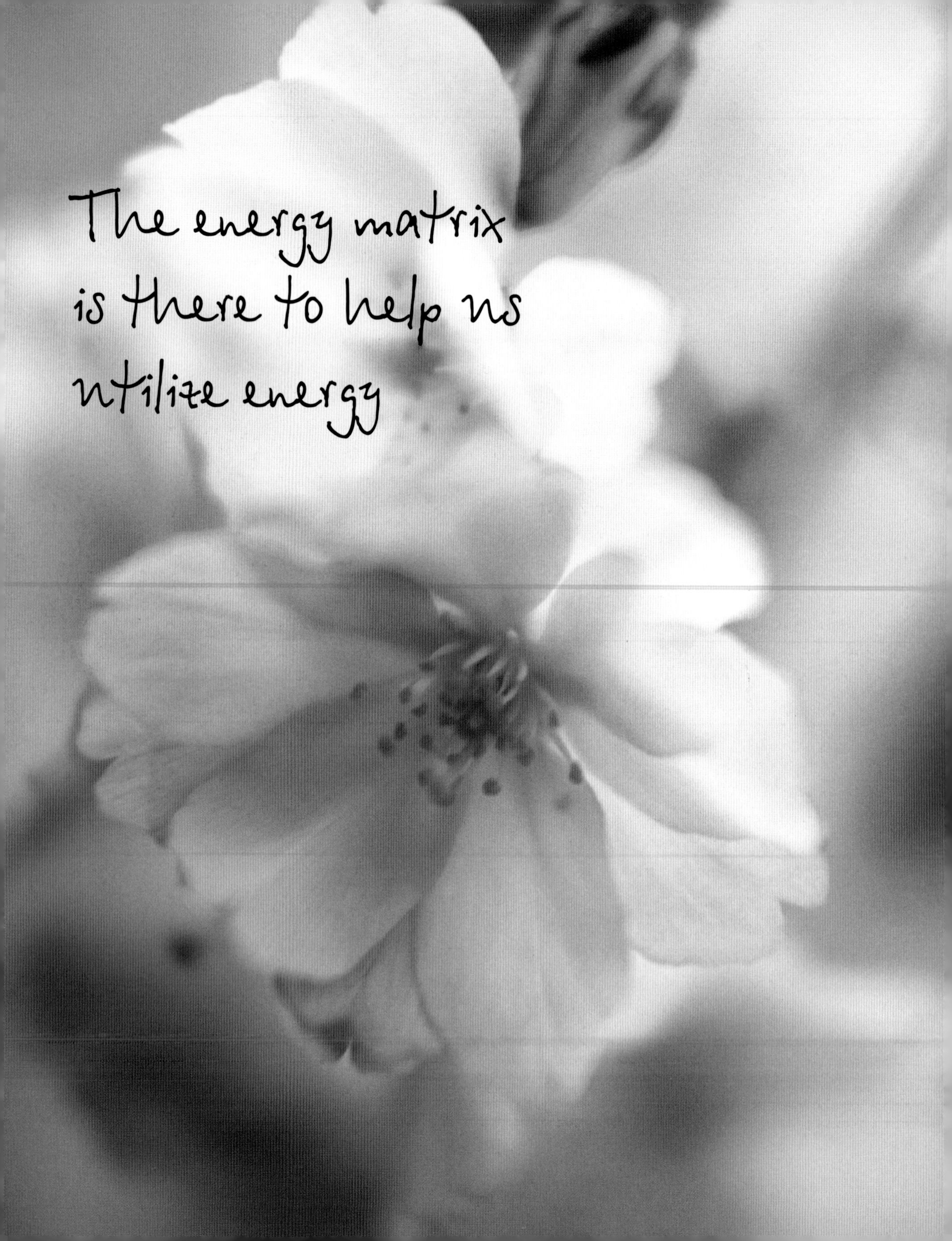

The energy matrix
is there to help us
utilize energy

own vibration – a word, sound, colour, picture, piece of furniture, letter – and, of course, flowers.

The history of your soul goes right back to the time you first evolved as a soul or spirit. I am not here to convince you of this – there are many wonderful books written by knowledgeable people and I have listed some further reading at the end of this book. However, I have first-hand experience of the validity of this statement since I have experienced spontaneous regressions myself, and seen them in my patients, and my work with soul retrieval, land clearing and house clearing cements this knowledge. So from the day we are born we have an old history and a new history trying to live side by side. Inevitably, sometimes, these histories are in conflict.

I've been playing with energy for a long time. In some ways I've been ignoring it, waiting for it to lose interest in me and go find someone else. Not to be, of course, I've now made the flower essence for *The Flower Healer*, Hard Seed Barb, and I'm facing yet more challenges head on. Sometimes I feel I've been dragged into the world of essences and energetic healing, and now into writing, but when I look at the bigger picture, I know that this is what I need and have to do.

When I started Essence World and opened the shop and clinic in Eton, I thought that was it – I would take essences to other people and help them see how they could change, as I had. I even read *The E Myth* by Michael E. Gerber, convinced I was not going to make the same mistake as countless others. I was divorced and settling into my new life, when I asked the question: How do essences really work? And I have been studying essences and energy ever since. I thought the end result was the shop, but it was only the beginning. My job now is to put what I know about energy and conventional medicine together and tie up how things go wrong – it's not difficult and doesn't have to be. Wow, was I ever wrong about my direction.

Energy is a product in its own right and the energy matrix is there to help us utilize energy – just as air is a product and our respiratory system is there to utilize it and help us to breathe. As a medium and clairvoyant, I have long had the ability to see the energy field as it truly is; I see the spiritual body and physical body linked by what I call the 'membrane'. This membrane is a fluid, rather viscous interface between the physical body and the spiritual body, and it receives, stores and utilizes information to keep the two bodies connected. This is where everything goes on and where it all falls apart when you are not true to yourself – it is the core of your vibrational energy or life force. Essences are the easiest way to work on your own vibrational energy – I believe they are the medicine of the future, the medicine of energy.

Above:
Sun Rose flower essence helps to strengthen our inner resolve.

Healing and the Chakra System

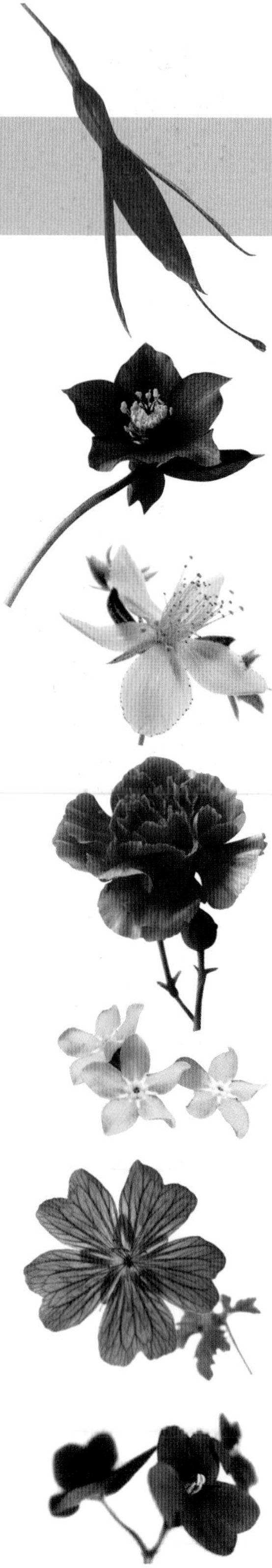

Originating in the Sanskrit language, the word 'chakra' means 'wheel', but I like to visualize a railway network, with each chakra representing a station. A railway system's sole function is to transport passengers and goods from A to B, whereas the chakras' function is to transmit messages from A to B. Each station, or chakra, has its own set of unique staff with specialized jobs and an infrastructure to support them. The train cannot move if there is no driver and fuel or electricity to move it forward, and in the same way messages cannot be delivered without impetus or indeed energy from substations or coils located around the body. These coils emit a strong energy, which acts as a magnet to the chakras and allows them to move in a circular motion or 'spin', very similar to the mechanics of a motor. These coils join forces around the body and, when healthy, unite and complete a circuit known as a matrix. This circuit must be complete to enable the chakras to spin freely and evenly – think of these coils as electricity substations, feeding the stations/chakras. When the chakras spin they also create their own energy, adding to the vibrational energy or life force being emitted.

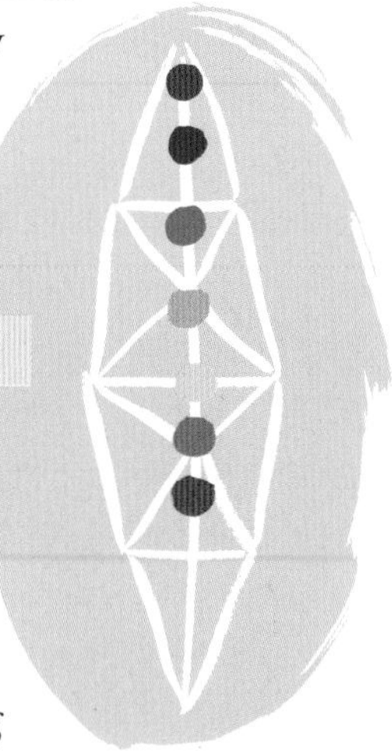

MATRIX WITH CHAKRAS

When we are born our matrixes are complete and work perfectly. There are two of them: one surrounding the physical body and the other the spiritual body. The coils then merge with their corresponding counterpart to bring these two bodies together, rather like two pieces of bread for a sandwich, while the filling is the membrane or the interface.

Crown chakra: violet/white
Third eye chakra: indigo
Throat chakra: blue
Heart chakra: green

Solar plexus chakra: yellow
Sacral chakra: orange
Base chakra: red

From the time of conception our chakras begin to mature. If you could see them with your physical eyes they would appear as little nipples similar to those on a cat and as we mature and grow, so do they. As our life unfolds we come up against many challenges: traumatic birth; first day at school; accidents; the many incidents that happen within our homes. We feel the shock of these episodes like ripples in a lake, permeating our many, many energy layers and components. The most important aspect of this shock is that our chakras are the only part of our energy field that is still growing and maturing, so a chakra will become damaged if it is going through a crucial part of its development when a shock happens – it is similar to taking a harmful drug at a critical stage of pregnancy.

So, to go back to the railway analogy, if we experience shock at about three years old, the base chakra will be affected. The amount of damage depends on the shock to the system – a worst-case scenario would be similar to a derailment on the line so the trains cannot come and go and passengers have to be ferried to other stations on buses and tubes. Some will not use the alternative transport and will put off their journey for another day. Others will have missed their appointment further up the track, so they go to their next appointment early instead, in another direction. In the same way, our chakras need to communicate their messages despite the malfunction, but in the chaos they have to find alternative routes, taking shortcuts or embarking on long out-of-the-way routes to achieve some form of communication. However, these routes already have their own functions, so they become burdened by the extra work and responsibility, until finally they wear out or become clogged and damaged themselves and it all becomes a bit of a mess.

The mature, healthy chakra should spin and open and close its lens at will, conducting the orchestra of sound within its structure and adding to the combined energy of the body, culminating in a 'life force' flowing within the entire energy body. The chakras receive energy from the earth, and this energy is then distributed throughout the body in various ways – ideally in a healthy and harmonious flow and pattern of interaction that encompasses all portions of the energy field, including the other chakras, the higher layers of aura, or energy field, and the organs and tissues of the physical body, and in other ways that support life.

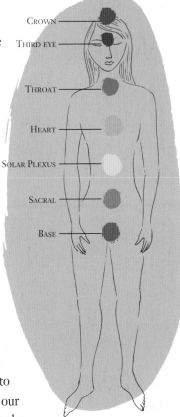

Above:
The seven principle chakras. The crown chakra alone is violet, but when all the chakras are working well together, the crown chakra turns white at the top.

Left:
The chakras are spinning wheels of energy, each with an associated colour.

The Flow of Energy

One aspect of this energy pattern is the upward flow of energy through the chakras. Beginning at the first or base chakra, there is a very significant energy flow that ascends through the chakra system – via the central energy channel in the spine – and continues to the seventh chakra. The lower chakras function in a simple way but the higher ones grow progressively more complex and spiritual. As the energy ascends through the chakras it is transmuted, or processed, by each one according to its nature, before continuing upward to the next chakra in the system. Like locks on a canal, each step takes the energy to a higher level than the step before.

Although this upward flow of energy is of primary importance, it is interesting to know that there is also a small but constant stream of energy flow back down the chakra system. Just like our railway system, trains arrive from other stations far and wide. The chakras connect with each other, yet each is like a small autonomous station, operating and running in accordance with its own particular nature.

In addition to their function as energy junctions, the chakras also have another important role. When not sending messages backwards and forwards they hum their own tune or radiate a chakra energy, each unique in its personality and function. Like families living next door to each other, they learn to live together and act as good neighbours and friends; when the street is cohesive it works as one and has a good energy. However, some streets have the 'neighbours from hell' so the energy is fragmented and shattered, and does not have a good feel. It is much the same with our chakras: when each one is contented and happy it radiates that energy outward from the body in a unique visual, energy field – which can be detected, by Kirlian photography, for instance.

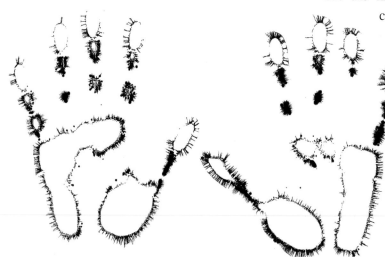

Above:
Kirlian photography captures a person's energy field, shown as 'spikes' around the forms of the hands and fingers.

Right:
Heliconium works on all levels of the base chakra and the matrix of the physical body, keeping the energy in place.

Dysfunctional Chakras

Each chakra vibrates to its own unique frequency or sound – the base chakra emits the lowest frequency and the seventh chakra the highest. Each chakra also vibrates to the same frequency as a colour; each colour represents a different frequency, rather like the colour coding system of electrical wiring. So each chakra has its own unique colour, corresponding to its place in the chakra system, and if the chakra is dysfunctional, blocked or broken, the colour is also affected. This discrepancy in colour is indicative of the overall state of the chakra itself and, like the derailment, it needs attention to prevent further damage to all the physical, emotional and/or mental bodies in the entire system. Many therapists use colour therapy in visualizations or meditations to help the chakra to achieve its potential, or to bring its colour back to a natural state. There are also many essences, such as Heliconium, that bring the individual chakra back into balance, hold it secure and allow the impurities to ease away, while maintaining the integral condition.

Unbalanced chakras have either too much, or too little, energy flowing through and within them. To understand this, let's go back to the example of the rail network. Say the 'derailment' has occurred at the second chakra: the result will be that, eventually, both the first and the third chakras are affected, because of the back-up of trains, or messages, waiting to get in and out. The first chakra (also known as the base, or root, chakra) is where we perform tasks relating to fear, security and stability, and sometimes the second chakra – which is responsible for our self-esteem – has to take over these functions. But its specialization is creativity and self-esteem, not fear, so chaos ensues because it is overworked and not performing the tasks it was meant for. The result is that we become over-aggressive, or retreating and non-confrontational because we want others to like us. Problems in one area of the matrix will always influence the operation of all other aspects of the energy field, to one degree or another. Dysfunctional chakras will unbalance your physical, emotional, mental and spiritual life.

Above:
Passion Flower helps to maintain the intrinsic energy of the body's life force.

Left:
Oriental Hellebore flower essence helps healing energy to flood through the entire chakra system.

Each of the seven chakras corresponds to a surrounding area of the body and affects the organs in its location.

CROWN (SEVENTH CHAKRA)	Hair and skin, pituitary gland, upper brain
THIRD EYE (SIXTH CHAKRA)	Eyes, ears, nose, head, pineal gland, nervous system
THROAT (FIFTH CHAKRA)	Throat, thyroid and parathyroid glands, mouth, teeth, gums, neck, vocal cords, jaw, shoulders, arms, hands
HEART (FOURTH CHAKRA)	Heart, lungs, thymus (immune system), circulation, vagus nerve, endocrine system, diaphragm
SOLAR PLEXUS (THIRD CHAKRA)	Adrenal glands, pancreas, liver, stomach, spleen, nervous system
SACRAL (SECOND CHAKRA)	Uterus, ovaries, bladder, kidneys
BASE (FIRST CHAKRA)	Bottom, rectum, spine, digestion and expulsion of waste, adrenals, bladder, hips, legs, feet

Above:
Each chakra relates to a specific part of the body.

As already mentioned, chakras can be damaged in many ways. Essences can help with energy problems, but bad damage may need manipulation by an experienced energy practitioner. Tears, breaks, even dislocation of the chakras need extra help – but fortunately they are uncommon.

Anne was diagnosed with schizophrenic tendencies, and was taking medication. She wanted a normal life, with a job and relationship, but had trouble integrating into new environments. Energetically, I sensed she had a very immature first chakra – my impression was it had stopped growing pre-birth. We set about encouraging it to grow, helping her deal with fear and insecurity from a stable foundation. As I explained this, she immediately asked, 'Do you think this could have anything to do with the fact that I was born without a uterus and vagina?' Of course, the two situations go hand in hand and although flower essences can't change the physical, we can change energetic problems. After one treatment, Anne volunteered for a job and is now thinking of training for a career. Directly after treatment, her lifelong friend noticed a positive difference, saying to her, 'Your energy has changed.'

Why Flower Essence Healing Works

Flowers, plants and trees have been on this earth for a very long time, and will doubtless exist for centuries well after we have gone. For thousands of years they have been used for their healing properties in therapies such as homoeopathy and aromatherapy, amongst others. Many people still confuse essences with essential oils. Aromatherapy is the art and science of using pure essential oils from plants for healing. Essential oils work through the subtle emotional body (a part of the

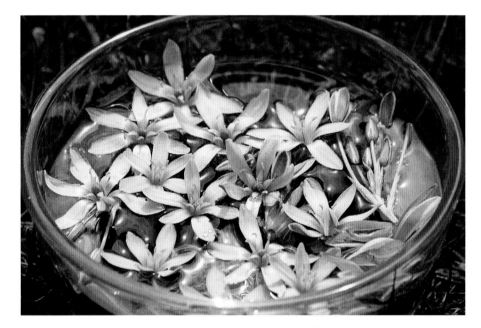

Left:
Making Star of Bethlehem essence by bathing the flower heads in a bowl of spring water.

aura) and the brain, where impressions of emotions and memory are retained. These essential oils are distilled or extracted by exerting pressure on fragrant plants, but flower essences are completely different.

Flower essences are generally made by floating flowers of the plant on spring water in a clear glass or crystal bowl in sun or moonlight, while calling upon the plant spirit (or deva) for the plant's permission and co-operation to use its energy in the essence. When making flower essences for healing purposes, nothing physical is transferred into the solution – the actual essence is the electromagnetic pattern of

I believe the
scope of healing
available through
flower essences
is truly miraculous
and ever-expanding

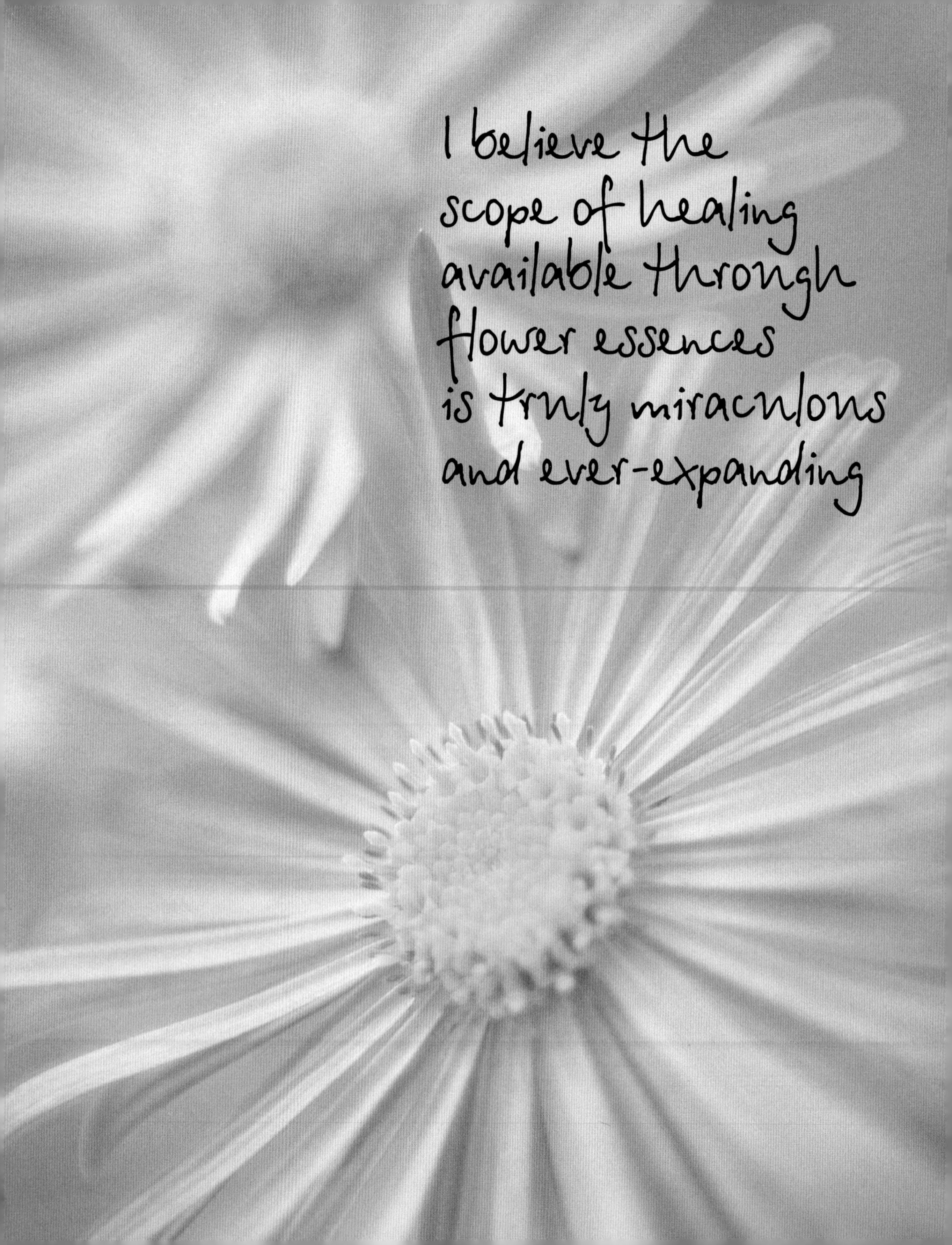

the flower. Just as there are nutritional elements found in plants that are useful for the health of the physical body, so there are patterns of biomagnetic energies discharged by the flowers on other frequency levels, which are useful for the health of your body's energy system. These are the life force – the highest frequency – of the plant, a bit like an electrical current. As flower essences are vibrational, they are also affected during their creation by the intention and energy with which they are made. Vibrational essences can also be made from crystals, gemstones, colours, sea and beach creatures, animals, and the energy of stars.

Above:
Because essences are vibrational, they can be made from virtually anything – from petals, leaves and bark to stone and shells.

I believe the scope of healing available through flower essences is truly miraculous and ever-expanding. Many essences work on an emotional level. They can encourage the purity of peace and serenity to replace the roller-coaster emotions we often experience in day-to-day living. There are essences that help us to face our fears with courage, rather than running away from them – there are even flowers to loosen old habits, clear depression and keep us walking on our divine preordained path, no matter what the obstacles.

Waking up your Energy

Flower essences represent a more harmonious way to clear and shift our energy field into higher states of vibrational purity. Many combination essences (two or more combined; see pages 84–87) allow for an even more powerful shift in the energy field. Various imbalances and toxins in the body are ultimately forced out because they are vibrating at lower frequencies – they don't vibrate at the level of health that flower essences propel us towards. Let's say, for instance, that I work at an optimum level when I have 240 volts charging through me, but that over a period of years some of my circuits have become worn out from too much work, or have fallen into disrepair because of neglect. Some of the leads and wires have so much dust from lack of care that they lie forgotten and idle, and this affects the total amount of energy I have available.

Imagine that you cannot use the bedroom in your house, because the lights won't turn on any more. So you start dumping boxes, junk, old giftwrap and broken furniture in there, because it's now effectively a spare room – one whole room wasted because it has no energy. In fact, you've forgotten you even had a bedroom; you're now sleeping on the couch. Essences have the ability to wake up that circuit from the inside, because they vibrate or 'hum'. The wires then vibrate to shake off the dust and are able to send out a clear sound. Once the infrastructure is working we can see that the problem is that the bulb has blown and needs restoring, so another essence is taken to revive the element in the light bulb and help it to heal. The light goes on, sneaking through the gap under the door and the next time you go past you think, 'Hey, what's that?' You had forgotten the room existed, but then you remember the mess that you left in there. Another essence later, and the next time you retire to your couch you remember the light, and the comforting, supportive feel of your bed, and you run upstairs to jump into a real bed. You spend the night sleeping fitfully, smelling the musty aromas of years of lying dormant, but in the morning you lean over and take your essence again and open the window.

Over time, and with the support of these wonderful essences, we become adept at activating those parts of ourselves so we will not need the flower essences as much. At first, though, it is best to take a little flower essence frequently, at least twice a day. Only a tiny bit of the flower's energy is needed to help shift us vibrationally and it starts to work instantly – but do bear in mind that if there have been years of neglect it may take you longer to recognize the changes.

Above:
Sun Orchid helps to stablize your ego.

Right:
Water Lily has a calming effect upon the nervous system and helps you to recognize the influences of truth and illusion.

Trust in your 'Self'

As a sensitive and a former nurse, I have a continual sense of awe about the relationship between the body and the spirit. As your heart opens, so does your intuition. Your intuition will teach you how to see and how to love. It will instil in you a renewed faith (in your 'self') to face anything in life. I feel that much could be done to prevent the soul wounding that takes place, if people could only be more conscious of just how their behaviour and thoughts can wound not only themselves but others.

We are the keepers of our own healing through our own insight (inside-looking). The only problem is that we have never learned this ability, or are clouded by other issues in our lives that prevent us from looking inside ourselves and seeing the answers. As a practising intuitive, my passion has been to bring spirituality and intuition into mainstream medicine. Then we can choose from the best of both worlds and, better still, mix the two. Intuition is the spiritual language that links us with our hearts, and thus to wellness. We can take a conscious viewpoint to be joyous and well. It is essential to develop positive beliefs about healing, a love for ourselves and an appreciation of the body's subtle energy system, and also learn to access inner guidance and listen to dreams. With these tools, we can maintain optimal health and be better equipped to face any health challenges that may arise.

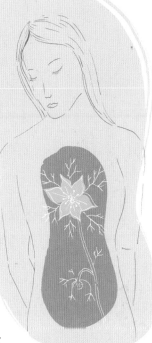

Is there a centre in our brain for spiritual experience? Scientists currently associate our spiritual centre with a part of the brain called the limbic system. When this area is electrically stimulated, some patients report visions of angels or devils. Likewise, if you smell the fragrance of your long-lost mother, you can instantly feel her embrace. It's powerful, this emotional stuff. Brain tumours, which overexcite the limbic system, can trigger enhanced spiritual awareness. What scientists are willing to conclude is that the brain and spirituality are interrelated; if you develop a belief in something greater than yourself, you will have a better chance of staying healthy longer, and a better chance of healing faster if you become ill.

Above:
Taking flower essences can help you heal from within.

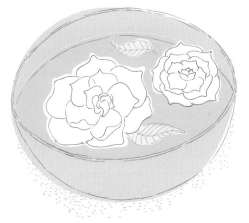

Chapter 2

How to Diagnose and Prescribe Flower Essences

Above:
Crocus helps you to overcome grief, loss and despair.

How does anyone prescribe or advise anything? They use their knowledge of the subject, weigh up the parameters of the issue, and make recommendations based on history, lifestyle, symptoms, desired outcome and efficacy. This rule applies whether you are a mechanic, PR consultant, doctor, dentist or business analyst. Sometimes you get it spot on, other times it may take round two to get to the exact solution. Perhaps one mechanic is better than the others, but why is this? You also have to take into account his history or knowledge – has he had previous experience with a Porsche, or does his main area of expertise relate to trucks? Does he ask you questions to prompt a memory of the symptoms? Is he listening and does he instil confidence? On the other hand have you, the customer, put your account of the problem into some semblance of order? Have you given an exact recollection of the symptoms to the mechanic? Maybe you've forgotten about that annoying little squeak whenever the brakes are applied. All these variables need to be taken into account.

When prescribing essences, either for yourself or others, variables such as these are also true, but a living being has one thing a motorized vehicle does not: emotions. When you recount your problem you try to state the situation as you see it. First mistake – sometimes your version of the truth is different from the real truth. When we are hurt we tell fibs to ourselves to help the pain go away. I have some patients (few, thankfully) who sit in front of me and lie – not only to me but also, more

Right:
Try to keep a note of your symptoms and which essences are effective for you.

harmfully, to themselves. They think, 'If I don't think about this, it will go away' and since that is what they want, they won't be honest. Or they will be embarrassed to admit things, so they leave them out or manipulate the truth. I had a partner who once said, 'I didn't lie to you, I just left out some "stuff"'. So, ask yourself, what 'stuff' do you leave out?

Left:
Geranium helps the soft side of sensitive individuals shine without fear of reprisals.

Choosing the Correct Essence

Before prescribing anything, tell the truth. Essences will only work if the correct essence is chosen. That doesn't mean you're never going to find the right essence – just that you have to be selective. Any one of us can look at most of the essences and say 'I need that one'. Of course, in some way we do, but do you need an inch of the cable unblocked or the whole length – and how many wires are crossing that blocked cable and are also affected? When we choose an essence our emotions naturally come into play – we avoid issues, dither and weigh up the pros and cons. Spending too long deciding affects our decisions, so I like the intuitive method because it's always right. In his book *Blink* (Penguin Books), Malcolm Gladwell talks about exactly this. 'Adaptive unconscious' is the power to make snap decisions and trust in the outcome. If we allow our other conscious self to make a decision, it always has an emotional slant. My Intuits™ system (see page 141) was developed with adaptive unconscious or intuition, and that's why it has had such phenomenal success, time and time again.

Below:
Dowsing with a pendulum is a very effective way to choose a flower essence.

However, as with any decision, you have to set your goals and decide what you want the outcome to be. Remember the car mechanic: what do you want your car to do? Do you know the problem is with the tyres, the engine, the radiator, or do you want a service to tell you what is wrong? On a personal level, is your question about moving forward, matters of the heart, do you need a good cleanse, or is there so much wear and tear you simply don't know where to start? Once you have decided this you are on the right path and your intention is clear. Now, and only now, start to track down your essence helper. Don't falter. Write your intention down and keep referring to it, as you will doubtless be swayed by the many options on offer. You can try opening this book at any page, then choose

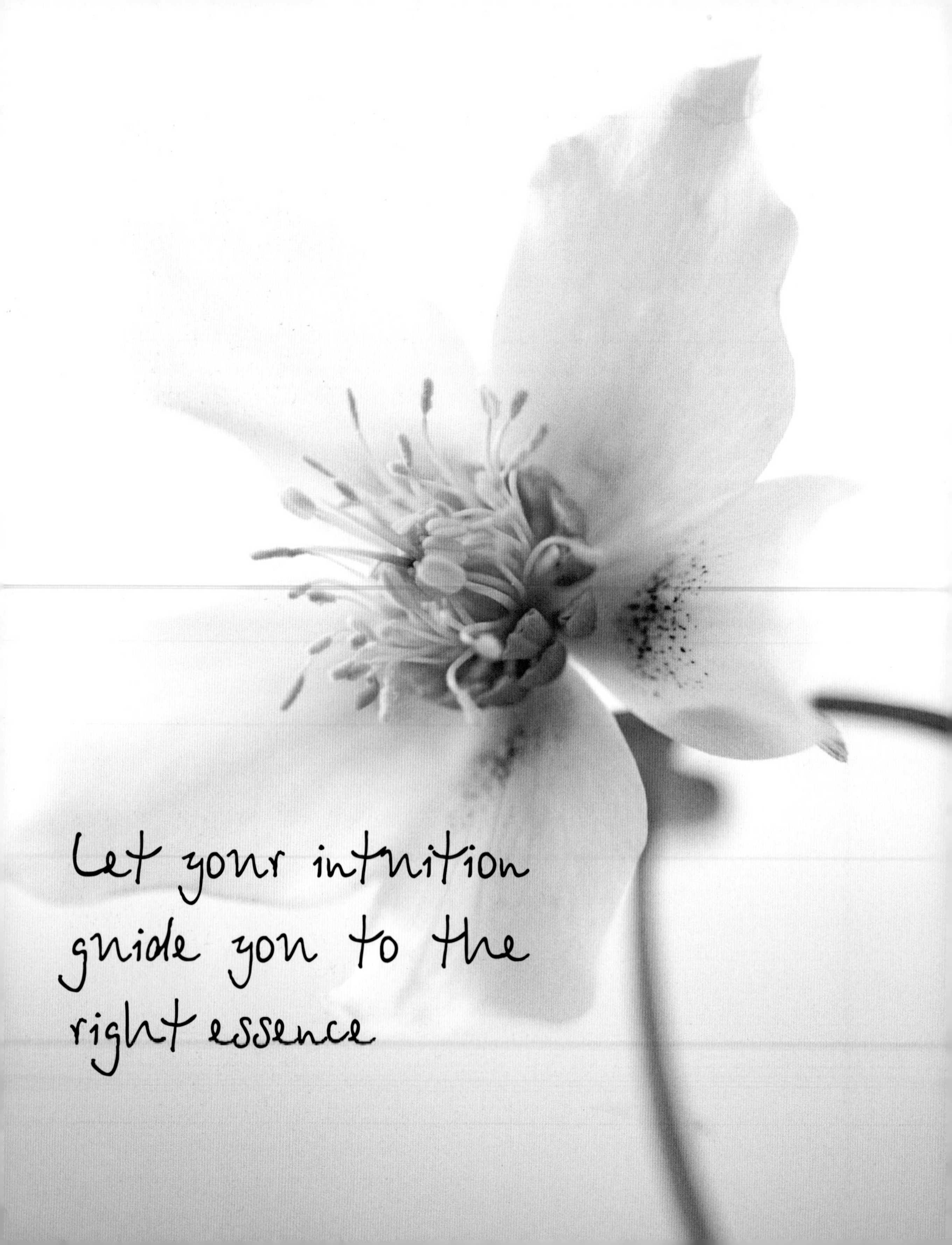

Let your intuition
guide you to the
right essence

either left or right, and, with your eyes closed, point to a place on the page and your essence will be written there. Or, use a pendulum, using the 'yes' or 'no' answer method with the question, 'Is this the right essence for these circumstances?' By using your intuition and keeping your intention firm, you will *know* the right one.

Alternatively, investigate the symptom finder. Draw three columns. In the first column, note down any symptom or illness you have at this moment; in the second, list anything you have had in the past; and in the third, anything you had as a child. Now start with the children's column, repeat your intention for the essence and choose a symptom you had as a child. Sound a little weird? Try it. I guarantee you'll find the cause right away. If you don't have anything in the third column, move to column two. Is there a pattern? Is everything fear-based, or is the majority of illness due to anger or lack of confidence? This works because you've eliminated your 'monkey mind', or the sound of your everyday thoughts, allowing your intuition, or adaptive unconscious, to answer.

If you want some expert advice, there are many knowledgeable and helpful essence therapists or practitioners for you to consult. A reputable flower essence therapist should talk with you for an hour and then suggest a single essence or blend of essences to take for a period, after which you come back for a follow-up session. I have worked like this myself, and it is successful, but for the past four years I have simply suggested a couple of essences and then let the client choose one or two themselves, because they know themselves more than I will ever know them. The results speak for themselves.

Above:
A chosen flower essence can be taken in many ways, such as adding drops to an unperfumed body lotion.

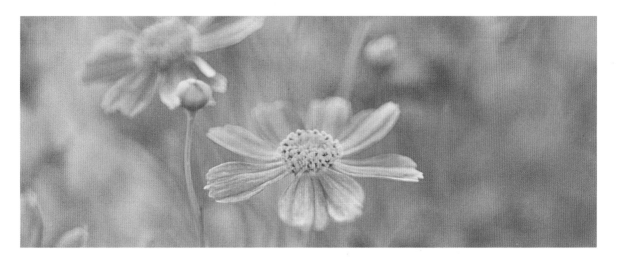

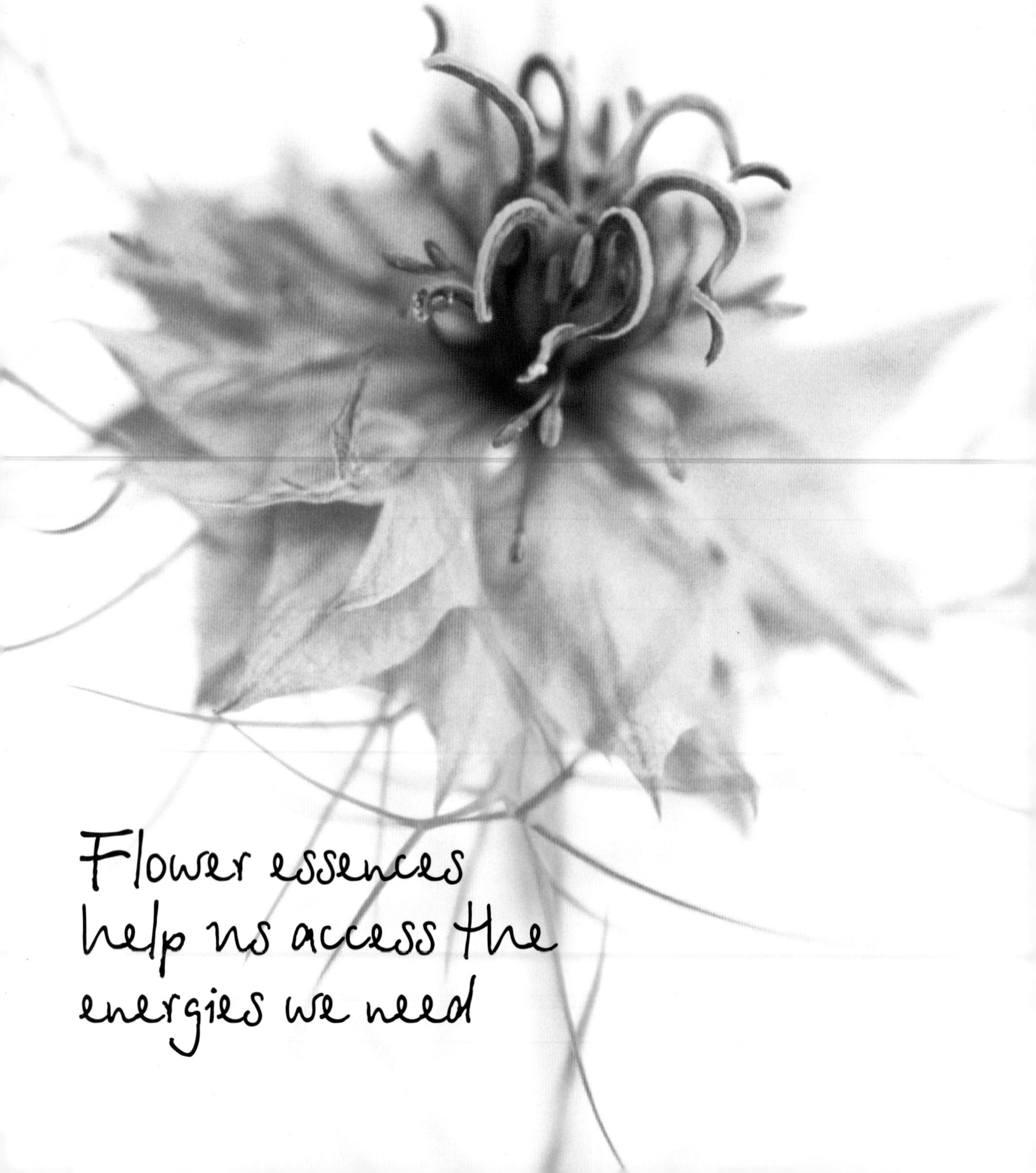

Flower essences
help us access the
energies we need

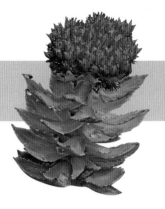

Chapter 3

Flower Essence Profiles

Flower essences help us access the energies we need, no matter what the season, or where we live in the world. Flowers, plants, trees and crystals have been with us a very long time, and their essences – or liquid energies – can help every one of us on our journey through life. It is said that even the plants in our garden are there specifically for us, and that we choose the house we live in because of the energy of the plants and trees in the garden. Take a moment to look at what is in your garden, and note which plants you are drawn to.

This is a selection of over 150 of the most chosen and used essences in my practice, including those from flowers and from some selected trees and crystals. The top twenty essences appear first, in order of their popularity. If you are thinking of investing in your own flower essences, these will form an ideal starter kit. The combined essences – those that comprise two or more essences – appear on page 137.

The essences are categorized into three groups: Leaders, Helpers and Mimickers. Leaders are bold, effecting change in your life whether you want them to or not; Helper essences are nurturing, helping to heal the energetic bruises, cuts and grazes acquired during the battles of the past; and Mimickers have the ability to mimic the helper or leader effect of any other essence they are mixed or given with.

Left:
Nigella damascena,
or Love in a Mist.

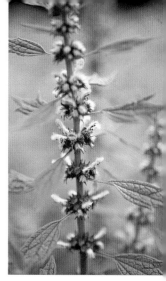

1 Magnolia *(Magnolia wieseneri)*
LEADER & MIMICKER

Country: Europe, America and Asia
Recommended source: Bodylink Essences

In Essence

This very feminine essence (yin) was made from a bloom that literally threw itself at my feet at the Westernbirt Arboretum, England. The huge flower has the most beautiful aroma, resembling that of Wintergreen, and even the essence has a slight scent. For centuries, organ makers have used the wood for valves and pipes. Similarly, Magnolia helps ensure clear energetic channels in the spiritual body. Use it for clarity, to stop procrastination, to stir intuition and develop a go-ahead attitude. It is the most commonly chosen essence in the Intuits™ system.

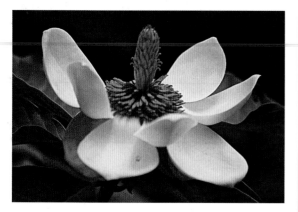

2 Motherwort *(Leonurus cardiaca)*
HELPER

Alternative names: Heartwort, Lion's Ear, Lion's Tail, Throw-Wort, Yi mu cao
Country: Europe, Central Asia, North America
Recommended source: Rising Serpent Essences, Illminster Essences

In Essence

Motherwort is a bitter, mint-like plant with a history of traditional uses as a mild sedative, calming agent and as

a treatment for epilepsy. The Latin *cardiaca* refers to Motherwort's traditional use to treat nervous heart-related conditions, such as palpitations and irregular heartbeat. The plant's active compounds include leonurine and stachydine, shown to lower blood pressure, treat anxiety and calm the nervous system. Motherwort essence is female (yin) energy and works on the intuitive crown to heart chakras, helping to eliminate negative cords and behaviour taught by your mother. Perfect for those with mothering issues, the essence brings a better balance in relationships, especially for an overprotective mother. It rebalances mind and body, creating peace and understanding. It may also help with hormonal imbalances, PMT and birthing issues.

3 Heliconium *(Heliconia caribaea* 'Black Magic') LEADER

Alternative name: Balisier
Country: West Indies, Colombia, Central America
Recommended source: Bodylink Essences

In Essence

This stunning plant flourishes in humid tropical rainforests. It loves light and so can grow to over five metres in order to reach the forest sun. A plantation worker in St Lucia first showed me the huge flower and I had to borrow a cooking pot to make the essence from a one-metre-high specimen! The essence was red when it was made and hot to touch. Energetically, Heliconium works on all levels of the base chakra and the matrix of the physical body, keeping the energy in place and enabling a secure environment from which to work. This essence is wonderful to use in times of fear and insecurity and to transform a slave mentality. It works with your 'fight-or-flight' response, helping you to fight or run as quickly as you can when appropriate, and it is one of the most commonly used essences in my practice. I really wouldn't know what to do without it.

4 Stargazer Lily (*Lilium orientalis*)
HELPER

Country: North America
Recommended source: Ilminster Essences

In Essence

The haunting aroma of the Stargazer Lily is recognizable as soon as you encounter it. The dreamy smell relaxes and creates the feeling of a private sanctuary, just like a desert island or a deep and cosy bed. The Stargazer Lily opens the pathway in the heart between the creative impulse, centred in the second chakra, and the sixth chakra (or third eye) through which creative vision moves out into the world. This essence doesn't increase creativity, but helps ease the bottleneck in the heart chakra caused by fear or lack of confidence. The Stargazer Lily allows energy to flow, increasing self-worth, love and positivity; it also helps improve performance at work or play. I prescribe it to help clients feel secure and connect with their inner wisdom.

5   Seaside Centaury
(*Centaurium littorale*) HELPER

Country : Europe
Recommended source: Ilminster Essences

In Essence

The harmonizing and calming effect of growing in sand dunes beside water allows this essence to be well grounded, connecting well with the Earth and the universe, and bringing about a better balance between the intellectual and the practical side of matters. Affecting the crown chakra, Seaside Centaury improves clarity. Use it for serious decision-making matters.

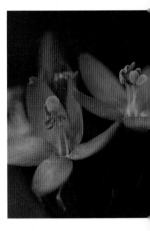

6 Betony (*Stachys officinalis Labiatae*)
HELPER

Alternative names: All Heal, Bishop's Wort, Common Hedgenettle, Heal-All, Lousewort, Purple Betony, Wood Betony
Country: Britain, Europe
Recommended source: Ilminster Essences

In Essence

Betony, a wild flower that grows abundantly in meadows and woodlands, is a member of the mint family and has been used medicinally since Roman times. The juice of the plant was frequently used to soothe headaches and heal cuts, ulcers and cold sores. It has become a popular remedy with modern herbalists for asthma, bronchitis and heartburn. As a flower essence, Betony relaxes the mind and triggers awareness of where true healing may lie or be required. It is powerfully restorative, but using it may mean that you reveal more to yourself and to others than you would like to admit. In my practice, this essence is commonly chosen by clients before an energy treatment, and certainly helps them to relax and talk about their concerns.

7 Passion Flower (*Passiflora bryonioides*)
LEADER

Alternative name: Cupped Passion Flower
Country: America (Virginia)
Recommended source: Rising Serpent Essences

In Essence

Sweet-scented and tinged with purple, Passion Flower is easily recognizable by its exotic fruit. Medically, its active constituent is passiflorine – a depressant with an effect similar to morphine. As a flower essence, Passion Flower helps to maintain the intrinsic energy of the body's life force. With this in place the major matrixes are working well. I have found that this essence releases tension around the heart area allowing a more relaxed relationship to blossom. It also relaxes the neck, which can help with breathing, and so relieve feelings of humiliation, grief and anger – usually aimed at the opposite sex.

8 St John's Wort (*Hypericum perforatum*)
LEADER

Alternative names: Goat weed, Hypericum, Klamath Weed
Country: Colombia, West Indies, Central America
Recommended source: Rising Serpent Essences
Combined essence: Lammas Goddess by Sovereignty Essences

In Essence

Commonly used in its herbal form to treat depression and anxiety, St John's Wort was also often traditionally hung over a picture to ward off evil – *Hypericum* is derived from the Greek *hyper* (above) and *eikon* (picture). This essence works with your 'fight-or-flight' response, helping you follow your instincts. Associated with the sun, the personality and consciousness, as an essence it is very helpful for dealing with father issues and for people lacking a strong sense of self and who are easily victimized. A fabulous essence for those quiet and shy types who both need and would like to be more assertive.

9 Christmas Cactus
(*Schlumbergera bridgesii*) HELPER

Alternative names: Holiday Cactus, Thanksgiving Cactus
Country: Brazil
Recommended source: Ilminster Essences

In Essence

The Christmas Cactus is a plant that grows above the ground – rooting into the decaying organic debris that is trapped among tree branches. It has flat, segmented, green leaves and blooms periodically, producing beautiful, long, pink, red, yellow and white flowers. By its very nature a tenacious plant, the essence of this cactus helps you to work your way through long-held emotional patterns that had seemed immovable, lifting each issue, one at a time, from the subconscious.

10 Lemon (*Citrus limonum*)
LEADER

Alternative names: Citronnier, Citrus medica, Leemoo, Limone, Limoun, Neemoo
Country: Northern India, Mediterranean
Recommended source: Sabian Essences

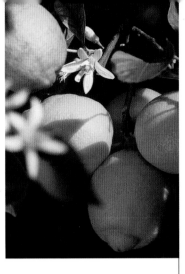

In Essence

The Lemon is a small, evergreen tree and gets its Latin name *limonum* from the Arabic *limun* or *limu*. Lemon is one of the best cleansers and astringents, and is said to be the most effective cure for severe, obstinate coughs. It is also helpful with jaundice and heart palpitations. As an essence, Lemon is an aggressive cleanser of the physical and spiritual bodies. It works deep in the bones, awakening and cleansing negative thoughts from all levels of the mind. Its sharp tang can unlock trauma associated with sexuality and relationship issues, working on the second chakra. The freedom this brings allows the mind to release, achieving peace and joy without blame or shame.

11 Geranium *(Geraniaceae)*
HELPER

Alternative names: Alum Bloom, Alum Root, Chocolate Flower, Crowfoot, Dove's-Foot, Shameface, Spotted Cranesbill, Storksbill, Old Maid's Nightcap, Wild Cranesbill, Wild Geranium
Country: Europe and America (Georgia, Missouri)
Recommended source: Sovereignty Essences, Korte Essences

Combined essence: Summer Solstice Goddess by Sovereignty Essences

In Essence

Geranium is an informal, cottage garden plant that is loved for its endless display of colour and for the divine aroma from its leaves when they are crushed, after the rain. Its aromatic oil is popularly used in aromatherapy for relaxing and balancing mind and body, and Geranium is a known astringent and tonic, having been used historically for the treatment of piles, diarrhoea, children's cholera, chronic dysentery and also as a good gargle. As a flower essence, Geranium is fabulous for sensitive individuals who are adversely affected by negativity. It says, 'Don't worry, be happy,' and can be used very effectively when another person is directing their negative energy onto you. This essence will allow their negativity to pass straight through the body – like Teflon for your energy field! Geranium can also be very effective on those affected by mass hysteria associated with fear.

12 Love in a Mist *(Nigella damascena)*
HELPER

Country: Europe, America, Australia
Recommended source: Rising Serpent Essences, Green Man Essences

In Essence

Quick-spreading Love in a Mist has been a popular garden plant since the 16th century. Perhaps it is its free spirit that makes it the perfect essence to create openness to loving and being loved. A very gentle flower essence, it works on the strands between the heart chakra and other, smaller chakras of the body and encourages you to be both strong and courageous. A physical cleanser, Love in a Mist also clarifies your emotional motivations, helping to ease frustrations and allow clear choices to be made. To calm and release old emotional trauma, this essence flushes the physical valve in order to clear any built-up debris from the physical body. Hurt and emotional pain can be effortlessly flushed away, leaving you free to create a more loving pathway.

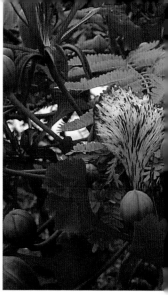

13 Blackberry *(Rubus fruticosus)*
LEADER

Alternative names: Bly, Bramble, Brambleberry, Bramble-Kite, Brameberry, Brummel, Bumble-Kite, Scaldhead
Country: Britain, Europe to the Mediterranean and Macaronesia, Australia
Recommended source: Bodylink Essences

In Essence

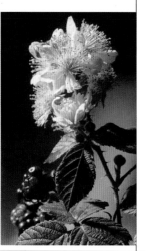

The humble Blackberry has a huge reputation as a charm and a medicine. The young shoots were believed to help secure loose teeth and the root-bark and leaves acted as a tonic and remedy for everything from dysentery to piles and cystitis. As an essence, Blackberry represents letting go – ideal when you feel you have no control over a situation and are unable to move through despondency, hurt, pain, and aloneness. Blackberry allows you to be yourself, helping you to manifest your desires where you have previously tried and failed. I also find the essence very useful for digestive problems, and it can help kick an addiction to adrenaline, bringing a semblance of order into your life.

14 Flamboyant Tree *(Delonix regia)*
LEADER

Alternative names: Peacock Flower, Royal Poinciana
Country: Barbados, Caribbean
Recommended source: Bodylink Essences

In Essence

This large umbrella-type shade tree has the most glorious flaming red blossoms. As an essence, it is ultimately about where you fit in life, about support and reassurance – for a conviction to survive the times, even though you feel stifled. It's for breaking free and testing the boundaries. Always supportive and supporting, my essence was made on the island of St Lucia in the Caribbean; the tree was entwined with a cabbage palm. I was drawn to the brilliant red flowers, but when I got a little closer, I noticed that there is always one white petal for every three red. Energetically this essence follows the adrenaline pathway, working on the top fifth of the base chakra, taking in the back portion of the second and just touching the base of the solar plexus.

15 Lamium *(Lamium maculatum* 'Chequers')
LEADER & HELPER

Alternative names: Dead Nettle, Spotted Nettle
Country: Britain, Europe
Recommended source: Bodylink Essences

In Essence

Rather ornamental for a nettle, Lamium has very pretty mauve-coloured flowers. Though unable to sting, its likeness to other nettles means it is generally mistaken for one and so is left alone by insects and humans alike. Like all nettles, Lamium is purifying for skin rashes and eczema and is used also homoeo-pathically. Energetically, Lamium can unwind chaotic energy around physical and spiritual bodies until clear

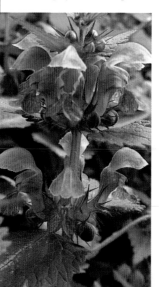

communication is possible. It is good for meditation, because it stops the chatter in your head. It is also very conciliatory; it allows all involved to see the same picture and do what has to be done without any thoughts of right or wrong. Lamium brings unquestioned trust, allowing you to initiate change at every level.

16 Mandrake *(Mandragora officinarum)*
HELPER & MIMICKER

Alternative names: Mandragora, Satan's Apple
Country: North Africa, Southern Europe
Recommended source: Sovereignty Essences
Combined essences: All blends by Sovereignty Essences

In Essence

The legendary Mandrake was believed to possess the magic power to heal a great variety of diseases, ward off evil and induce a feeling of love and happiness; its roots were once as expensive as gold. In my experience, Mandrake essence is most effective when placed on top

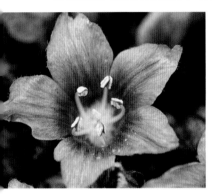

of the head. It creates a very strong link with the levels of awareness that interface with the human, plant and spirit worlds. It clarifies reasons for emotional outbursts, increases dynamism and energy, and allows visionary flow and creative ideas.

17 Star of Bethlehem
(Ornithogalum umbellatum) HELPER & MIMICKER

Alternative names: Bath Asparagus, Dove's Dung, Sleepydick, Star of Hungary, White Filde Onyon
Country: Europe, Mediterranean
Recommended source: Bodylink Essences, Bach Collection by Sun Essences

In Essence

Found in grassy meadows in Europe, this pretty star-like white flower is known as one of the five key essences in Dr Bach's calming Rescue Remedy. The fresh plant is toxic though the bulbs are edible and can be roasted like chestnuts. Star of Bethlehem works on the physical energy body to release tension. Shock causes us to take a sharp intake of breath; holding it

creates a rush of adrenaline trapping the trauma of the incident in our physical tissues, so they contract, which in turn can create pain – both physical and emotional – but Star of Bethlehem allows this tension to subside. It is very useful for those suffering with addictions. For knocks and scar tissue add a few drops to your favourite cream and gently apply.

18 European Spindle Tree
(Euonymus europaeus) HELPER

Alternative names: (French) Bonnet-de-prêtre or Fusain d'Europe, Burning Bush, Dogwood, Fusanum, Fusoria, Gadrose, Gatten, Gatter, Indian Arrowroot, Pigwood, Prickwood, Skewerwood, (German) Spindelbaume, Wahoo
Country: Europe
Recommended source: Sovereignty Essences
Combined essence: Samhain Goddess by Sovereignty Essences

In Essence

Found in hedges and copses, this smooth-leaved shrub bears loose clusters of small greenish-white flowers. The rose-red fruit bursts when ripe to disclose ruddy-orange seeds wrapped in a layer of scarlet flesh. The plant acts as a tonic and, in small doses, stimulates the appetite and gastric juices. As an essence, it energizes the soul, and accesses the energies of the shadow-self (your dark side – the naughty bits) but in an integrated, positive way. By promoting an understanding of your true nature and needs, it dispels feelings of inferiority or superiority, and allows an increased sense of security, reducing the need to compare yourself with others.

19 Mexican Tarragon (*Tagetes lucida*)
HELPER

Alternative names: Pericon, Sweet Mace, Texas
Tarragon
Country: Mexico, Guatemala (Sierra Madre Oaxaca
Mountains)
Recommended source: Sovereignty Essences
Combined essence: Samhain Goddess by Sovereignty
Essences

In Essence

This cousin of the better-known French Tarragon is
more vigorous and easily grown in warmer climates. It
can be used in the spicy dishes that are popular in its
place of origin and is sometimes added to pot pourri
and flavoured vinegar. With a sweet, anise flavour, it
makes a lovely addition to soup, while the pretty yellow
flowers are a nice surprise to pep up a salad. It has also
been used to make a tea for hangovers and to relax both
nerves and stomach – it seems to have similar
properties to Peyote, so the stronger the tea the more
europhic you become. The stronger version, *yauhtli*,
was most probably used by the ancient Aztecs in human
sacrificial ceremonies – along with the petals, which
were added to resins to be burnt as incense – helping
the victims to go voluntarily to their death.
Historically, the Aztecs also used Mexican Tarragon as
a medicine for their physical ailments. It is no surprise
that the essence is known for its ability to clear
thoughts and for astral travel, helping to keep the
energy of the body stable whilst travelling through
other dimensions, and is also good for therapists who
use their powers of clairvoyance to help the client.

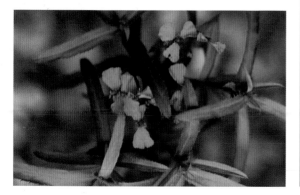

20 Pine (*Pinus sylvestris*)
HELPER & MIMICKER

Alternative name: Scotch Pine
Country: America
Recommended source: Bodylink Essences (Helper), Soul
Quintessence System (Helper & Mimicker), Bach
Collection by Sun Essences
Combined essence: Heart to
Heart by Bodylink Essences

In Essence

Most Pine trees have straight,
unbranched, cylindrical trunks,
and all Pines yield resin; it is
mostly used to create oil of
turpentine, for soap-making and
medicinally for ointments,
plasters and inhalants. Likewise,
in its essence form, Pine clarifies
everything. Direct, straight and
focused (like the tree), Pine
essence brings awareness, which
is the first step to change. By
being aware before venturing,
you may say: 'Don't go down
that road.' Clear perception also

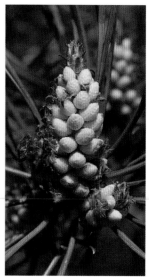

allows you to see that the cup is either half-full or half-
empty, depending on your perspective. Pine clears,
bathes and protects the mind, creating a focused mind-
to-heart connection. It helps the mind to look beyond
failure, guilt, loss, ridicule, or the other traps that would
have you avoid lessons or address them in a superficial
way, which would rob you of deeper experiences. Pine
assists you in working through life's lessons and taking
those experiences to a new level of understanding. It
helps you to make conscious choices and to release
symptoms such as restlessness (moving from one situation
to another with no real purpose), avoiding responsibil-
ities, inability to connect life experiences at a soul level,
being out of tune with the rhythms of nature, keeping the
mind busy to cheat yourself of inner reflection, and
impatience regarding your own or others' slow progress.
You can also use Pine essence for headaches caused by
stress, sleeplessness, loss of balance, an overactive mind,
narrow-mindedness and scattered thoughts.

Lady's Smock (*Cardemine pratensis*)
HELPER

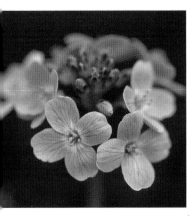

Alternative names: Cuckoo Flower, Milkmaid
Country: Britain, Europe
Recommended source: Bodylink Essences
Combined essence: Peace Nostrum by Bodylink Essences

In Essence

A pretty flower, Lady's Smock looks a little like a pinky-lilac buttercup. In Europe, much superstition surrounded this flower; it was believed that if anyone picked it, a thunderstorm would break out and it was also thought to generate lightning so it was never taken into a house. In parts of England the plant was believed to attract adders, Britain's only poisonous snake, and it was thought that anyone picking it would be bitten before the year was out. The essence reflects the fact that the plant is immersed in tradition, most importantly in relation to the family. Use Lady's Smock for a better understanding and awareness of family history and the part it has to play in your own development as an individual.

Snowdrop (*Galanthus nivalis*)
LEADER & HELPER

Alternative name: Milkflower
Country: Switzerland, Austria, Southern Europe
Recommended source: Rising Serpent Essences (leader), Green Man Essences (helper)
Combined essence: Demeter – Hope by Gaia Essences

In Essence

Named *Galanthus*, Greek for 'Milkflower', the Snowdrop – as one of the earliest flowers in the year to blossom – is among nature's optimists. Its healing properties were known as far back as 1465 – an active substance in Snowdrop may help treat Alzheimer's Disease. As a flower essence, Snowdrop works on the throat, heart and solar plexus chakra – allowing energy to run unhindered with force from the universe. It creates a surge of energy in the chest to give the momentum to move forward from 'issues'. It can be taken when you're feeling frustrated or just worn down. It also helps those who have become withdrawn from their sexuality due to abuse, because it reveals the hidden beauty and strength within and can create a spiritual breakthrough.

Lilac (*Syringa vulgaris*)
HELPER

Country: Persia, Europe, Africa
Recommended source: Soul Quintessence System
Combined essence: Auric Shield

In Essence

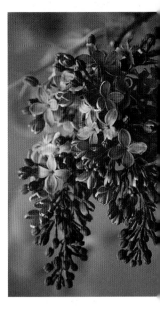

The pretty, scented Lilac, easily recognized by its boughs of tiny pyramidal flowers, has been used in medicine to reduce fevers and in the treatment of malaria. As a flower essence, Lilac works on over-sensitivity, inflammations, psychic attacks and negative thought patterns. It reinforces the aura, cleansing debris out of its various layers, and neutralizes the effects of old trauma in the subtle bodies. Once emotions are released and cleared, Lilac increases stamina and strengthens the immune system. Lilac essence is cool and soothing on burns. Lilac may also be helpful in places with fluorescent lighting and computer equipment and in areas where high levels of pollution tear at the aura, making it a travel essential.

Oriental Hellebore *(Helleborus orientalis)*
LEADER

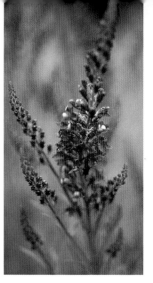

Alternative name: Lenten Rose
Country: Eurasia, including Greece, Turkey, The Caucasus
Recommended source: Sovereignty Essences
Combined essence: Imbolc Goddess by Sovereignty Essences

In Essence

The Oriental Hellebore is an attractive little evergreen that is especially valued for its fine foliage and for its attractive blooms. Its shy flowers resemble single roses but nod their pretty faces toward the ground. They are long-lasting and remain beautiful as they slowly fade. Healing energy floods through the entire chakra system with Oriental Hellebore essence, which reduces tension, over-energy and over-excitability. It also increases self-assurance and reduces shyness, thereby encouraging self-awareness, poise, clarity and balance. Use it to help re-establish your direction and goals in life.

Purple Toadflax *(Linaria purpurea)*
HELPER

Alternative names: Aaron's Beard, Climbing Sailor, Creeping Jenny, Ivywort, Mother of Millions, Mother of Thousands, Oxford-Weed, Pedlar's Basket, Pennywort, Rabbits, Roving Jenny, Thousand Flower, Wandering Jew
Country: Britain, Europe (Mediterranean)
Recommended source: Ilminster Essences

In Essence

The plants of Purple Toadflax send up dozens of metre-high flower spikes, covered in tiny purple, pink and white flowers that bumblebees find irresistible. In Italy it is the 'Plant of the Madonna'; it prevents scurvy and is used in India for diabetes. With a smell similar to cress, it has also been eaten in salads across Europe for years. I love this plant – it makes the bees happy, seeds itself with wild abandon filling empty spots in the garden and makes a great flower essence for inner wisdom (the third eye). Perfect for when you need to face a block in life, this essence replaces irritation and blindness with patience and observation, especially when there appears to be no obvious answer to an issue, a situation, or life in general.

Forget-Me-Not *(Myosotis arvensis)*
HELPER

Alternative name: Field Forget-Me-Not
Country: Northwest Africa
Recommended sources: Sovereignty Essences, Green Man Essences
Combined essence: Beltane Goddess by Sovereignty Essences

In Essence

Forget-Me-Not is the quintessential English wildflower, creating a vision of blue mist carpeting woodlands when its dainty flowers bloom. As an essence, the flower brings about awareness of karmic connections in your personal relationships and the spiritual world. Mindful of subtle realms, it integrates the crown chakra activities of meditation, dreams and visions. Take Forget-Me-Not essence to boost mental agility and clarity of thought and to release negativity. Perfect for those with soul isolation, who lack the awareness of a spiritual connection with others and consistently block off communication from other dimensions.

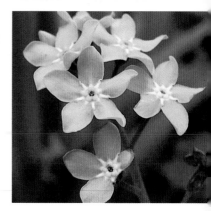

Tobacco Plant (Nicotiana 'Lime Green')
HELPER & MIMICKER

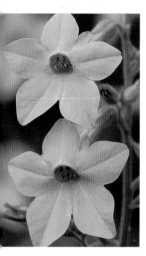

Alternative name: Tabbaq
Country: America (Virginia), China, Europe
Recommended source: Gaia Essences
Combined essence: Demeter – Hope by Gaia Essences

In Essence

The huge leaves of the Tobacco Plant grow freely; they are slightly hairy, pale green in colour, with a narcotic odour, and a nauseous, bitter taste. Tobacco is, of course, an irritant, causing violent sneezing when chewed; in large doses it produces nausea, vomiting, sweats and weak muscles. However, medicinally it is used as a sedative, diuretic and expectorant and internally as an emetic. As a plant essence Tobacco is all about joining in – perhaps this reflects the very social art of smoking, although of course this is now a dying trend. Take it if you are on the lookout for joy and happiness; it will help to put you into the situation rather than standing back like a wallflower. It is helpful for children and adults alike who desperately want to join in and have fun, but just cannot find the strength to do so.

Italian Arum (Arum italicum)
HELPER

Alternative names: Adder's Root, Arum, Bobbins, Friar's Cowl, Kings and Queens, Lords and Ladies, Parson and Clerk, Quaker, Ramp, Starchwort, Wake Robin
Country: Southern Europe, Britain (Isle of Wight)
Recommended source: Soul Quintessence System
Combined essence: Insight

In Essence

Arum starch was used for stiffening ruffs in Elizabethan times and the French still use the stalks of the plant as a soap substitute. In essence, too, it's about strength and clarity: when you rely heavily on the knowledge of others, rather than seeking it from within. Whenever you feel spiritually blocked, Arum connects you with divinity, strengthens your inner voice and generates the confidence, know-how and enthusiasm to act on it. Therapists and healers will find this essence very useful for providing accurate messages. It is also supportive during meditation and clearing sessions; it may be used to clarify vision, bring understanding, activate the third eye chakra, and pinpoint long-standing issues. Italian Arum helps us realize that God is in the hearts of all.

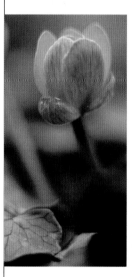

Marsh Marigold (Caltha palustris)
HELPER

Alternative names: Bull's Eyes, Horse Blobs, Kingcups, Leopard's Foot, Meadow Routs, Solsequia, Verrucaria, Water Blobs
Country: Britain, Europe
Recommended source: Bodylink Essences
Combined essence: Peace Nostrum by Bodylink Essences

In Essence

The flower of the Marsh Marigold resembles a gigantic purple buttercup. With almost hollow stems, it is often found in wet meadows and by streams. The English name Marigold refers to the Virgin Mary; an alternative, Verrucaria, comes from its ability to cure warts; Solsequia was given because the flower opens at the rising of the sun and closes at its setting – this may account for Marsh Marigold's amazing ability as an essence to help balance sleep patterns. It 'shines a light' on dark situations and helps shift-workers improve their sleep patterns. Since there's little doubt that we all feel more content in ourselves after a good night's sleep and some sunshine, Marsh Marigold reflects this too.

Oak (*Quercus robur*)
HELPER

Alternative names: Common Oak, Tanner's Bark
Country: Britain, Europe, America, Mexico
Recommended source: Bodylink Essences, Green Man Essences, Soul Quintessence System, Bach Collection by Sun Essences
Combined essence: Heart to Heart by Bodylink Essences

In Essence

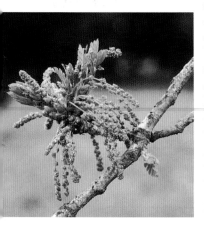

The mighty Oak has been the chief forest tree of Great Britain for centuries, intimately bound up in its history since the Druids. Its medical action is slightly tonic, strongly astringent and antiseptic. Like other astringents, Oak has been recommended for agues (alternating shivers and fever), haemorrhages, chronic diarrhoea and dysentery and it is a very good substitute for Quinine in intermittent fever, especially when given with Chamomile flowers. As an essence, Oak can 'get to the root of the problem', helping you understand the purpose and meaning of your roots, earthly and celestially. Oak helps you recognize that family beliefs and social conditioning can support or obstruct your development. It allows you to release any tension that arises in personal and global relations, preserves crucial knowledge and helps you realize the meaning of true unity – which is to be aware and open to your needs, the needs of others and the environment. Ultimately you need to remember where you come from, who you are and what you hold within. Being out of sync with your real roots may result in over-sensitivity, weakness of character, attachment to limiting beliefs, narrow-mindedness and being judgemental. Oak encourages the soul to speak in its natural form and it may be used to strengthen the nervous system, combat over-sensitivity and fatigue, and to ground you when you're feeling spaced out.

Ajuga (*Ajuga reptans*)
LEADER & HELPER

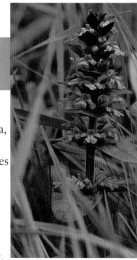

Alternative name: Bugle
Country: Europe, Britain, North Africa, Asia, Australia
Recommended source: Bodylink Essences
Combined essence: Peace Nostrum by Bodylink Essences

In Essence

Medicinally, the leaves of the Ajuga plant are both a diuretic and stimulant. Ajuga was highly regarded in the treatment of rheumatism and also women's menstruation problems. A tonic to the system, cleansing and purifying, Ajuga is about communication, bringing clarity and focus to the mind. I use this essence to help verbal communication, allow compromise and reach an acceptable outcome for all. With the intricate throat chakra cleared, Ajuga then allows energy to flow through the shoulders and arms so it can be helpful for problems such as a frozen shoulder.

Hazel (*Corylus avellana*)
LEADER

Country: Europe, Britain
Recommended source: Green Man Essences, Sovereignty Essences
Combined essence: Imbolc Goddess by Sovereignty Essences

In Essence

The name Hazel is derived from the Anglo-Saxon *haesel knut* – *haesel* meaning cap or hat, referring to the cap of leaves on the nut when it is on the tree. The male and female flowers of this small, hardy type of birch both grow on the same plant; the male yellow catkins open like drooping 'lamb tails', while the female flowers appear as tiny pink tufts on plump buds and will later turn into hazelnuts. The Celts associated the

Hazel tree with wisdom and poetic inspiration and it was thought that new skills and knowledge could be gained by eating hazelnuts. The tree is also a symbol of fertility. A Hazel rod is said to protect against evil spirits and was the best twig for water divining, while hazelnuts were carried as charms or to ward off rheumatism. Hazel essence helps to boost your cross energy and enhances the ability to receive and communicate wisdom. It clears away unwanted debris and brings stability and focus, allowing you to integrate useful information – making it great for all forms of studying. I think of it as 'the flowering of skills'. Interestingly this debris is released from the soles of feet, so when taking it try walking barefoot in the grass – or if you live near the sea, walk at the water's edge – to release it back into nature.

Baobab *(Adansonia digitata)*
LEADER

Alternative names: Bottle Tree, Dead-Rat Tree, Monkey Bread Tree, Upside-Down Tree
Country: Africa
Recommended source: Rising Serpent Essences

In Essence

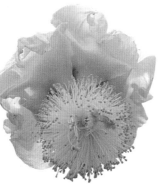

The huge Baobab tree bears big, heavy, white flowers and its large, gourd-like, woody fruit contains a tasty pulp that dries, hardens and falls into pieces that look like chunks of dry bread. Baobab essence reflects the power of this mighty tree, and can strengthen the very foundation of your physical body. Working on the coils of the physical matrix and the pathway into the physical body, the essence works on the kind of very deep-seated trauma that can sometimes render you incapacitated – such as trauma caused by war or child abuse. It heals deep wounds and may also help with addictions, psychosis and other traumas.

Primula – Yellow *(Primula vulgaris)*
HELPER

Alternative names: Artetyke, Arthritica, Buckles, Cowslip, Crewel, (*Anglo-Saxon*) Cuy lippe, Drelip, Fairy Cups, Herb Peter, Key Flower, Key of Heaven, Mayflower, Our Lady's Keys, Paigle, Palsywort, (*Greek*) Paralysio, Password, Peggle, Petty Mulleins, Plumrocks
Country: Britain, Europe
Recommended source: Bodylink Essences
Combined essence: Peace Nostrum by Bodylink Essences

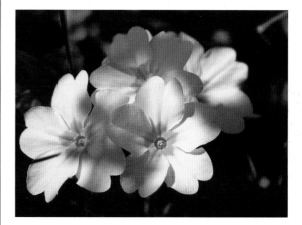

In Essence

An ancient and well-loved wild flower, Primula's alternative name of Cowslip is believed to come from a corruption of 'Cow's Leek' – leek is derived from *leac*, Anglo-Saxon for plant. In pagan times it was called Herb Peter and Key Flower, because the pendant flowers looked like a bunch of keys, the emblem of St Peter. The flowers have a very distinctive, fresh fragrance and slightly narcotic juices, which have led to the making of Cowslip wine as a sedative. Hugely popular in home remedies, Cowslip flowers were also believed to help strengthen the nerves and the brain, relieving restlessness and insomnia. In an essence, Primula attracts positivity from people and success – all the right vibes. By balancing and increasing your energy to attract other positive energies around you, this lovely little flower relieves depression and leaves the way clear to transform an ugly duckling into a beautiful swan.

Yarrow – White (*Achillea millefolium*)
HELPER

Alternative names: Bad Man's Plaything, Bloodwort, Carpenter's Weed, Devil's Nettle, Devil's Plaything, Field Hop, Herbe Militaris, Knight's Milfoil, Milfoil, Nose Bleed, Old Man's Pepper, Sanguinary, Soldier's Woundwort, Staunchweed, Thousand Weed, Yarroway
Country: Britain
Recommended source: Gaia Essences
Combined essence: Mary – Purification by Gaia Essences

In Essence

Yarrow grows everywhere, sometimes becoming a troublesome weed. The plant has downy stems and an attractive cluster of white or pale lilac flowers. Yarrow was formerly much esteemed as a wound healer and Gerard tells us it is the plant with which Achilles staunched the bleeding wounds of his soldiers, hence the name of the genus, *Achillea*. It was once dedicated to the Evil One and in earlier days was used for divination in spells. An astringent, tonic, and stimulant, Yarrow tea is a good remedy in the early stages of a child's cold. In essence form, Yarrow offers protection – use it to help keep personal boundaries free of others. It is perfect for the victim and those who are easily influenced by the thoughts and deeds of others.

Bakul Tree (*Mimusops elengi*)
LEADER

Country: India
Recommended source: Soul Quintessence System
Combined essence: Sacred Shield

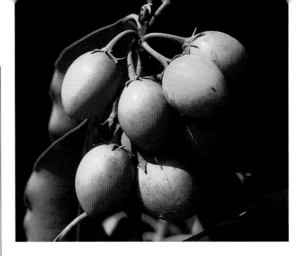

In Essence
The sacred Bakul Tree adorns many an Indian temple courtyard with its deep green leafy boughs. Its exotic flowers look spectacular and smell truly divine. Endowed with religious symbolism, the Bakul Tree has a vast pharmacy of remedies, utilized for centuries for ailments ranging from sore muscles and the common cold to malaria and epilepsy. Bakul flowers are still used as temple offerings to please the gods and are worn as garlands at festivities. So imagine all that in an essence: close your eyes and expect to be released and cleared from religious dogma, fanaticism, separation, or being self-opinioned or cut off spiritually. The Bakul Tree is all about realignment, remembrance, miracles of creation, openness, communion and sacred truth.

Verbena (*Verbena bonariensis*)
HELPER

Alternative names: Purple Top, Vervain
Country: America, Southern Europe
Recommended source: Gaia Essences
Combined essence: Athena – The Warrior by Gaia Essences

In Essence

The upright and rather wiry stems of this form of Verbena carry tufts of tiny purplish-blue flowers. This plant is very popular in mixed borders or flower beds because the tall, thin, see-through stems allow the flowers to be produced without concealing those growing behind. This is also a plant that attracts butterflies – including painted lady and meadow brown,

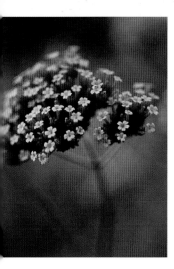

as well as the hummingbird hawk moth – and it will self-seed where it is happy without any fuss. The name Vervain is thought to be derived from the Celtic words *fer*, to remove, and *faen*, stone, referring to its use in treating bladder stones. As a flower essence, Verbena creates that 'can do, will do' attitude, and enables you to turn negative apathy into positive action.

Blue Iris (*Iris versicolor*)
HELPER

Alternative names: Blue Flag, Dagger Flower, Dragon Flower, Flag Lily, Liver Lily, Lunar Blue Iris, Poison Flag, Snake Lily, Water Flag
Country: North America, Canada
Recommended source: Ilminster Essences

In Essence

Blue Iris or Blue Flag was once one of the most popular medicinal plants amongst various native North American Indian tribes. In modern herbalism it is mainly employed to detoxify the body by increasing urination and bile production. It has a mild diuretic and laxative effect and when taken internally as a tea the dried root acts strongly on the liver and stimulates the circulatory and lymphatic system. Its detoxifying effect makes it useful in the treatment of psoriasis, acne, herpes, arthritis, swollen glands and pelvic inflammatory disease. Blue Iris works on the solar plexus and I find it unblocks spiritual talents of knowing and expression. But use this essence with care – it is very powerful and may bring up deep emotional issues that need to be dealt with.

Sun Orchid
(*Epidendrum chioneum*) HELPER

Country: Australasia
Recommended source: Korte Essences

In Essence

The Sun Orchid gets its name from its habit of remaining closed except in strong sunlight. This Tasmanian plant has been steadily decreasing in number, so it is now listed as an endangered species. Precious indeed, Sun Orchid essence helps to stabilize your ego. It offers protection to your physical body, helping it to balance and repair by increasing the overall cross energy. It fosters the ability to stabilize and repair, so the solar plexus is given the impetus to move; it opens and connects to the sun and the life-giving elements of solar power.

Wych Elm (*Ulmus glabra*)
HELPER

Alternative name: Scotch Elm
Country: Britain, Europe, North and West Asia
Recommended source: Green Man Essences

In Essence

Wych Elm is a tall tree with drooping branches and smooth, thin bark. As a tonic, astringent and diuretic, elm has been known to treat ringworm and a homoeopathic tincture is used as a cleanser. In essence, it works from crown to root chakras, ensuring a constant energy-flow, easing emotional blockages, shifting obstructions and flowing around them. Gentle in its approach, it brings the mind swiftly to clarity. With a life-affirming outlook you achieve peaceful awareness and a new-found confidence in personal strengths and abilities.

Water Lily (*Nymphaea alba*)
HELPER

Alternative names:
Sweet Water Lily,
Water
Nymph
Country:
Britain, Europe
Recommended source:
Soul Quintessence
System

In Essence

The Water Lily represents a peaceful
retreat from this mad world. The
rhizome eases pain, while the root
treats dysentery, bronchial catarrh
and kidney pain. The flowers have a calming effect upon
the nervous system and are useful in treating insomnia.
Water Lily essence helps you to recognize how truth
and illusion influence your life and pinpoint the real
issues to understand whether your motivation is fear or
inner knowing. Underachievement, lack of purpose,
fault-finding and blame, seeing only the bad in others
or focusing on the dark aspects of life may have blurred
your vision, but Water Lily lights the way to truth and
crisis management, helping you to seek a higher state
of awareness and share this understanding with others.

Foxglove (*Digitalis purpurea*)
LEADER

Alternative names: Bloody Fingers, Dead Men's Bells,
Fairy Caps, Fairy's Glove, Fairy Thimbles, (*German*)
Fingerhut, Folk's Glove, Gloves of Our Lady,
(*Norwegian*) Revbielde, Virgin's Glove, Witches' Gloves
Country: Britain, Europe, Madeira, The Azores
Recommended source: Bodylink Essences

In Essence

The Foxglove is a favourite flower of the honeybee. As
he moves from flower to flower up the spike, pollen is
rubbed off his back from one blossom to the next and

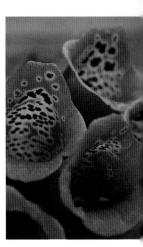

hence the flower is fertilized. First
called Folksglove – the glove of the
'good folk', or fairies – the mottlings
on the blossoms, like the spots on
butterfly wings and on the tails of
peacocks and pheasants, were said to
mark where elves had placed their
fingers. Today, the Foxglove is
cultivated to provide the drug
digitalis for heart complaints – it
increases the activity of all muscle
tissue, especially that of the heart,
arterioles and circulation. Foxglove
essence strengthens the heart, too: originating from the
base chakra, it follows the energy line of the vagus
nerve, filtering through every tiny strand of the physical
body. Foxglove essence focuses the inner ear to hear
what the heart is truly saying. A true tonic for the
emotions, it is ideal for the person who has been hurt in
childhood and has not been able to voice their pain – yet!

Sun Rose (*Cistus albidus*)
HELPER

Alternative names: Canadisches
Sonnenroschen, Frostplant,
Frostweed, Frostwort Cistus,
Helianthemum Ramultoflorum,
Rock Rose
Country: Southwest
Europe, Mediterranean,
North Africa
Recommended source:
Korte Essences

In Essence

Sun Rose is a small evergreen shrub
with whitish leaves that grows in rocks
and, like all the *Cistus* family, its pink or purple flowers
only last a day but keep on coming. Sun Rose essence
works on the base chakra and all etheric levels. It
strengthens your inner resolve so that you remain
centred and able to persuade others in a group to
follow you. Use it for confidence, especially at times
when you lack self-assertiveness or backbone.

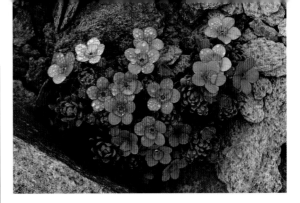

Alder (*Alnus glutinosa*)
LEADER

Alternative names: Red Alder, Smooth Alder
Country: America, Europe
Recommended source: Green
Man Essences

In Essence

A well-known shrub, growing in clumps by ponds or rivers, the Alder bears both male and female flowers. Medicinally, Alder is a tonic, astringent and emetic, and it has a bitter taste. The inner bark of the root is emetic, and the cones that grow on the bark are boiled to make a decoction which is said to be astringent, and useful in many types of haemorrhages. As an essence, Alder gets to work in the core of the body to assimilate the flow of energy. It increases the flow of vibrational energy, brings clarity of mind and eases stress. I often use it in my practice to reduce nervousness and anxiety.

Rock Jasmine (*Androsae occidentalis*)
HELPER

Country: East Asia (Himalayas from Sikkim to Kashmir)
Recommended source: Bodylink Essences
Combined essence: Peace Nostrum by Bodylink Essences

In Essence

A hardy plant that can grow at high altitudes, Rock Jasmine requires rock garden conditions in full sun to thrive at sea level. The entire plant has long been used in Tibetan medicine for the treatment of disorders, from all kinds of tumours to inflammations. It has a bitter taste and a cooling effect and as an essence, it tells you to dry your tears. It says, 'Enough is enough, honour the pain and move on'. Don't put the issues facing you in a box and lock the lid – keep the lid off and don't hide or shy away; look them square in the face. A great leveller, Rock Jasmine helps the body to avoid storing negative emotions inside.

Knotgrass (*Polyganum aviculare*)
HELPER

Alternative names: Allseed, Armstrong, Bird's Tongue, Centinode, Cowgrass, Hogweed, Nine-Joints, Ninety-Knot, Pigrush, Pigweed, Red Robin, Sparrow Tongue, Swine's Grass, Swynel Grass
Country: Britain, Europe
Recommended source: Silvercord Essences

In Essence

A common weed in grassland, Knotgrass is abundant everywhere you look, its woody root taking a good strong hold of the earth. Old herbals call it Bird's Tongue or Sparrow Tongue, due to the shape of its small, pointed leaves. Its minute reddish flowers also gained it the name of Red Robin. The plant cools, cleanses and heals and has astringent and diuretic properties, making it useful in treating kidney infections, diarrhoea, bleeding piles and haemorrhages. Energetically, Knotgrass works on all levels of the chakra system stemming from the solar plexus, increasing energy into the smallest of threads and nadis. Used mainly as an essence for stomach problems and also for the joints, remember it when you need to be flexible and bend in certain situations.

Wild Cherry (*Prunus avium*)
LEADER

Country: Britain, Europe, North Africa, West Asia
Recommended source: Green Man Essences

In Essence

The Wild Cherry has attractive clusters of white flowers followed by round red fruit and the tree is noted for attracting wildlife. The plant is self-fertilizing – the flowers are hermaphrodite with both male and female organs and are pollinated by bees. The fruit stalks are astringent, sedative, diuretic and a tonic and are used in the treatment of cystitis, oedema, dyspepsia and anaemia. The plant is useful for chest problems, particularly bronchial complaints, catarrh and whooping cough. An aromatic resin can be obtained by making small incisions in the trunk, which has been used an inhalant in the treatment of persistent coughs. As an essence, Wild Cherry stops cross energy and allows the body to channel a smooth flow of energy, allowing you to focus on the emotions. It focuses energy in the physical body and stimulates self-healing.

Similarly, Wild Cherry essence calms the heart and mind and is useful where there is extreme emotional pain.

Ceanothus (*Ceanothus*)
HELPER

Alternative names: California Lilac, New Jersey Tea
Country: North America
Recommended source: Gaia Essences
Combined essence: Isis – Divine Understanding by Gaia Essences

In Essence

A beautiful shrub with a vast number of small, blue flowers, Ceanothus is astringent, antispasmodic, and a sedative used to treat asthma, chronic bronchitis, whooping cough and dysentery. Working on the throat chakra and on the issues held in the vibrational energy system, including the thyroid, Ceanothus essence is all about your soul identity and the development of unconditional love. The first thing a newborn encounters on this planet is the reality of its existence. This may cause deep trauma, a sense of isolation and loss of confidence later in life, and a feeling of 'I don't want to be here'. Take Ceanothus to negate these feelings – whatever your age.

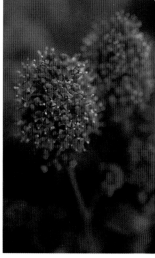

Dianthus (*Dianthus plumarius*)
HELPER

Alternative name: Pinks
Country: Britain, Europe, Asia, Africa
Recommended source: Gaia Essences
Combined essence: Isis – Divine Understanding by Gaia Essences

In Essence

Dianthus are the quintessential cottage garden flowers. Superbly scented, they're extremely easy to grow and add a lively summer touch to the garden. Some varieties of Dianthus have been grown for centuries – they were first brought to Britain in the 11th century by Norman monks and can still be seen clinging to castle ruins – and by their nature, Dianthus often rejuvenate by reseeding themselves. In essence, Dianthus is perfect for those times when you are suffering from physical fatigue and your body simply wants to stop. You will suddenly get this incredible burst of energy – like an alarm clock it wakes you up, feeling revitalized, as the Dianthus says 'enough time asleep, let's get on with it'.

Roseroot (*Rhodiola rosea*) HELPER

Alternative names: Burnirot, Golden Root
Country: Newfoundland, Europe, Asia
Recommended source: Silvercord
Essences

In Essence

For centuries Roseroot
has been used in
traditional medicine in
Scandinavia and Russia,
treating depression,
fatigue and anaemia. In
the mountain villages of
Siberia a bouquet of roots
enhances fertility and assures the
birth of healthy children. Needless to say, as an
essence, Roseroot helps to balance the mind, body and
spirit, and is great when you need to connect to life's
purpose, and for self-love. It works by increasing
receptivity in your physical and spiritual coils and helps
the chakras to spin in perfect harmony.

Orange Azalea (*Rhododendron austrinum*) HELPER

Alternative names: Florida Azalea, Rhododendron
Country: America (Florida, Georgia)
Recommended source: Ilminster Essences

In Essence

Each year, for several weeks at a time, Orange Azaleas
dominate the landscape with their breathtakingly
brilliant golden blossoms. The showy flowers are
golden yellow trumpets, often blushed red or peach at
the base, and produce a delightful honeysuckle-like
fragrance enjoyed by butterflies, hummingbirds and
humans alike. Working on the heart chakra, Orange
Azalea essence symbolizes 'Love Unlimited'. A very
important essence, it allows cosmic love to flow into
and through the heart, embracing self-forgiveness, and
melting deep irritations and old hurts. I find this

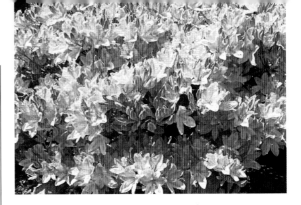

essence is chosen over and over again by adopted
children, however old, and if this is your story you
may want to add this to Olive for a perfect balance.

Blue Spiraea (*Caryopteris incana*) HELPER

Alternative names: Bluebeard, Blue Mist
Country: America, Britain
Recommended source: Ilminster Essences

In Essence

This brilliant vivid blue flower, with its clusters of
aromatic, velvety petals, loves the sun, attracting bees
and butterflies in wild abandon. In essence, Blue Spiraea
acts like a 'virus check' for the body's computer, helping
to dissolve attached, imbalanced energy patterns. Picture
it as if there's something in your make-up that has you
repeatedly following certain bad habits or negative
family traits, or falling for the wrong man or woman,
every time. Likewise, maybe the energy of someone
around you has his or her hooks into you – and every
time they think of you, it pulls at you. Sound familiar?

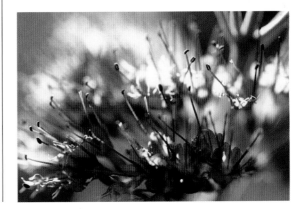

Ash (*Fraxinus excelsior*)
LEADER

Alternative names: Common Ash, Weeping Ash.
Country: Britain, Europe, North America
Recommended source: Green Man Essences

In Essence

The Ash is a fast-growing, tall, strong, handsome tree, famous for its tough yet flexible wood. The bark treats rheumatism, liver disorders and fever; the leaves have diuretic and purgative properties. There are many old superstitions concerning the Ash; typical is its reputation for magically curing warts. Understandably, the essence is perfect for balancing any discord within the body. It helps you feel flexible, secure and 'in tune'. Cross energy is amplified, sight is more focused and there is harmony all round.

Rowan (*Sorbus aucuparia*)
HELPER

Alternative names: (*Irish*) Caorthann, (*Gaelic*) Caorunn, (*Welsh*) Cerddin
Country: Britain, Europe (Iceland to Spain)
Recommended source: Soul Quintessence System

In Essence

Easily recognizable by its distinctive leaf, the Rowan is a vigorous-growing, hardy, deciduous tree. As a plant essence, Rowan is for remaining flexible; for moving through your growth cycles without trying to control life's sudden twists and turns. Rowan addresses issues such as excessive ambition, indecisiveness, stagnation or complacency. Beneficial for those who are disillusioned with their personal and spiritual development, Rowan helps you to acknowledge the stepping-stones that enable you to reach your purpose safely. Trusting in divine direction can be a truly liberating experience, opening the way to purer consciousness. Use Rowan to balance the nervous and vascular systems or when a crisis – such as puberty, pregnancy or grief – occurs.

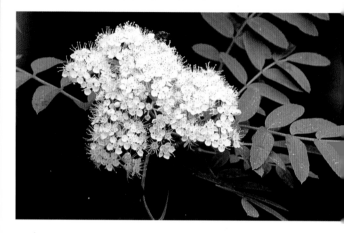

Agrimony (*Agrimonia eupatoria*)
HELPER

Alternative names: Church Steeples, Cockeburr, (*Anglo-Saxon*) Garclive, Philanthropos, Sticklewort
Country: Britain, Europe, North America
Recommended source: Ilminster Essences

In Essence

Known to all country-folk, Agrimony has a reputation as a medicinal herb. The graceful, slender spikes of yellow flowers, which have a refreshing, sweet aromatic 'apricot' scent, were once brewed up to purify the blood. Modern herbalists still value the herb as a mild astringent, tonic and diuretic. Its essence works on the base chakra as the pacifier. Often referred to as the 'light bringer', it inspires spiritual awareness and wisdom. Use it to gain courage to face situations – a strong stomach – and to 'face your demons' in any area of life that you may be avoiding, and ultimately to give balance and courage in whatever it may be necessary to face.

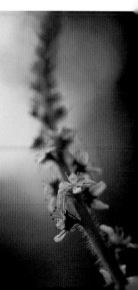

Viburnum (*Viburnum tinus*)
HELPER

Alternative name: Laurustinus
Country: Southern Europe, Britain
Recommended source: Sovereignty Essences
Combined essence: Winter Solstice Goddess by
Sovereignty Essences

In Essence

This common form of hedging – which is actually from
the same family as the honeysuckle, though it doesn't
smell nearly as nice in wet weather – is extremely
tolerant and adaptable to most soils and heavy pruning.
As a flower helper, the essence offers support and
reassurance if you feel unsettled, vulnerable or unhappy.
It helps to establish identity and direction, particularly
after life-threatening traumas and situations.

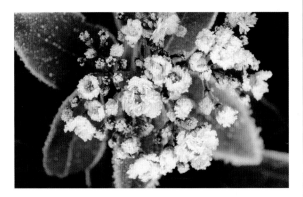

Quaking Grass (*Briza maxima*)
HELPER

Alternative names: Great Quaking Grass, Rattlesnake
Grass
Country: Mediterranean, Channel Islands
Recommended source: Silvercord Essences

In Essence

Mostly found on dry, hot banks, basking in the
sunlight, this distinctive, ornamental grass has compact
flowers and seed heads that gracefully nod and shake on

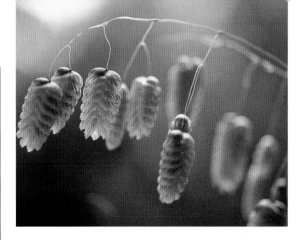

their stalks in the breeze. In essence too, Quaking
Grass will help you to be strong of heart and overcome
nervousness. Great for bringing subconscious issues to
the fore, it gives more protection over the heart and
solar plexus. This means that instead of nodding your
head in agreement just to keep the peace, you feel
stronger and better able to stand up for your rights.

Musk Orchid (*Herminium monorchis*)
HELPER

Country: Britain
Recommended source: Silvercord Essences

In Essence

Musk Orchid is a tiny plant that is pretty hard
to spot until you recognize its minuscule,
bright, yellow-green flowers, glowing amidst
the lime of abandoned chalk quarries. The
flowers have a strong honey scent (not
musk) that is deeply alluring to equally tiny
insects. Sadly, the ploughing-up of old
grassland has resulted in the demise of this
species in many areas and it is also highly
sensitive to drought. Musk Orchid
essence works on the solar plexus and
the heart. Like a gentle vacuum cleaner,
it draws out debris from the physical
coils. It acts on the mental emotional
bodies by enhancing mental structure to overcome
rigidity and by dissolving blockages. I have also found
Musk Orchid essence alleviates the conscious or
subconscious fear of being touched. Repeat this
affirmation, 'I bring peace to every part of my being.'

Wormwood (*Artemesia absinthum*)
LEADER & HELPER

Alternative name: Green Ginger
Country: Europe, Siberia, Britain, America
Recommended source: Sovereignty Essences
Combined essences: Lammas Goddess and Autumn Equinox Goddess by Sovereignty Essences

In Essence

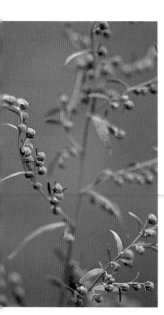

Although one of the bitterest herbs in existence, Wormwood is very wholesome and was reputed to counteract the effects of poisoning by Hemlock and toadstools. Absinthe, a tonic for the nerves, soothes spinal problems and calms the nerves. An excellent remedy for poor digestion, loss of appetite, and for preventing sickness after meals, Wormwood essence can help to release fear and anxiety from the second and third chakras. It can give empowerment, determination and the desire to take control over your life once more.

Golden Rutilated Quartz
HELPER

Alternative names: Sagenite, Venus-Hair Stone
Country: Tanzania, Madagascar, Brazil, South Africa, India, Sri Lanka, Germany, Switzerland
Recommended source: Gaia Essences, Soul Quintessence System
Combined essence: Solaris by Soul Quintessence System

In Essence

Golden Rutilated Quartz contains small titanium oxide crystals that arise at high temperature and pressure and become trapped inside the quartz crystals as they cool. As well as making the quartz rare and costly, the rutiles magnify its healing and spiritual properties. An important healing stone, Golden Rutilated Quartz integrates energy for cleansing and energizing the soul, filtering out negative energy and removing barriers to spiritual growth, making it ideal for when you need to change direction in life. It soothes dark moods, offering relief from fears, phobias and anxieties by working on all the chakras to strengthen the flow of energy used to communicate with the brain: think of it acting as a positive radar to pick up higher energies. Take it to realign soul power, inner strength and lightness of being. Use it to physically aid respiratory problems and cell regeneration. It is also an excellent balancing stone for a sad or weak heart.

Lime – Citrus (*Citrus aurantifolia*)
LEADER

Alternative names: Bartender's Lime, Key Lime, Mexican Lime, West Indian Lime
Country: Southeast Asia, West Indies, Mexico, America (Florida, Texas, California)
Recommended source: Sabian Essences

In Essence

The zesty, fresh flavour and aroma of Lime has made this small fruit popular for flavouring drink. The small shrubby tree has many thorns, and in colder climates can be grown in conservatories in the winter – the tree needs warmth to create the best fruit. Valued as a citric essence for its amazing cleansing ability, Lime essence affects all the layers of the physical body for a better balance. It is much softer than Lemon in its action, more centred on emotional cleansing, and is anti-stress.

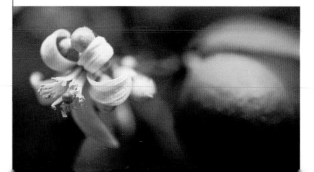

Bay Cedar (*Suriana maritima*)
LEADER

Country: America
Recommended source: Bodylink Essences

In Essence

Coastal habitats are among the harshest environments, and many plants in these locations develop thick, stiff

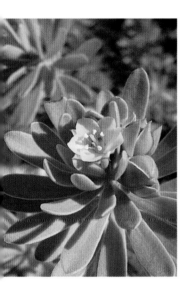

leaves, or armour themselves with thorns. Not so the Bay Cedar, a gentle shrub seemingly out of character with the austere locale – yet it thrives tenaciously. As an essence, Bay Cedar is all about protection. It allows you to grow, unaffected by the negative environment around you. Acting like a cloak, Bay Cedar protects and stabilizes even in the roughest storms, allowing the jewel of light within you to shine. Essential if you work in the City.

Yew (*Taxus baccata*)
LEADER

Country: Europe, North Africa, Western Asia
Recommended source: Green Man Essences, Rising Serpent Essences
Combined essence: Winter Solstice Goddess by Sovereignty Essences

In Essence

No tree is more associated with legend than the Yew. Sacred to the Druids, the association of the tree with places of worship still prevails. The wood was used for making longbows – it is said to resist the action of water and is very hard. Although highly toxic, Yew has occasionally been used medicinally. Modern research

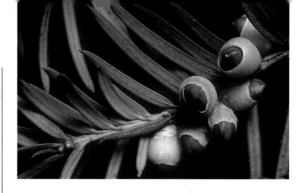

has shown it to contain taxol, a potential as an anti-cancer drug, in its shoots. All parts of the Yew, except the fleshy fruit, are antispasmodic, expectorant and purgative and have a beneficial effect on the heart. The leaves have been used in the treatment of asthma, bronchitis, and epilepsy, and also been added to a steam bath as a treatment for rheumatism. Energetically, Yew essence increases the strength and vitality of the spiritual coils for a deeper connection. Helping you to *see* the real situation, it increases cross energy at the very base of the body, and protects you from harm by activating the highest spiritual values of survival and protection. Take this essence to energize the body, sharpen the memory, and boost the body's defence system.

Victoria Regia (*Victoria amazonica*)
LEADER

Country: Brazil
Recommended source: Korte Essences

In Essence

This famous giant flower opens at night only to close again in the morning trapping unwary insects inside. When the flower reopens, releasing the insects to pollinate other buds, it has changed colour from creamy white to dark pink. In essence, Victoria Regia works by letting light into the subconscious and opening valves. This essence contains energy related to the Kundalini, which considerably improves your physical condition and also helps those of us who are on the threshold of leaving this world and going into the next.

Fuchsia (*Fuchsia magellanica*)
HELPER

Alternative name: Hardy Fuchsia
Country: South America
Recommended source: Gaia Essences
Combined essence: Athena – The Warrior by Gaia Essences

In Essence

A robust, hardy plant, this Fuchsia has pretty pinky-red and purple flowers that are produced in abundance in season. The flower often attracts hummingbirds for pollination, but it can vary from white to dark red, purple-blue and orange. The fruit is a small, edible berry which has a subtle peppery grape flavour. The 'look at me' aspect of the Fuchsia is reflected in the essence, which is all about wanting to change a low opinion you might have of yourself. The people and circumstances around you often reflect what you don't like about yourself; Fuchsia helps to unblock emotions and allows truth to blossom by opening up the heart chakra, so you can recognize these patterns in yourself, then let go and change.

Cedar Sunset (*Cedrus atlantica*)
LEADER, HELPER & MIMICKER

Alternative name: Atlas Cedar
Country: Morocco (Atlas Mountains), Algeria
Recommended source: Cedar Sunset by Bodylink Essences

In Essence

The Cedar is a large, majestic evergreen conifer with silvery grey bark, and stiff, needle-like bluish green leaves. An essential oil obtained from the distilled branches makes an effective antiseptic and fungicide that stimulates the circulatory and respiratory systems and also calms the nerves; it is also astringent, diuretic,

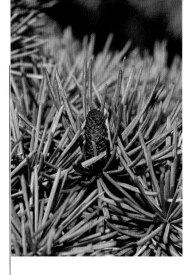

expectorant and sedative. Diluted with almond oil, and massaged into the skin, it is used in the treatment of skin diseases, ulcers, chest infections, catarrh, cystitis and dandruff. Used as an inhalant it treats bronchitis, tuberculosis and nervous tension. By a process of increased diffusion, Cedar essence helps to release the 'energetic waste' that coats the spiritual and physical valves through the main core of the body, passing them into the membrane or water element of the body for filtering. The essence cleanses thoughts that can keep you separate, alone and aloof. Because it cleanses without acknowledgement it is lovely when added to a night-time dose, helping you to process during sleep, when the body is resting, and allowing you to sleep restfully. It is particularly effective when the chest is congested and it is more difficult to sleep.

Thistle (*Cirsium vulgare*)
HELPER

Alternative name: Common Thistle
Country: Britain, Europe (from Scandinavia south and east), North Africa, West Asia
Recommended source: Soul Quintessence System
Combined essence: Communion

In Essence

The common Thistle is a pernicious weed that spreads freely because its seed can be dispersed by the wind over large areas of grassland. The flowers attract wildlife and are pollinated by bees, flies, moths, butterflies and beetles. A hot infusion of the whole plant has long been used as a herbal steam treatment for rheumatism and to treat bleeding piles. Energetically, Thistle essence works from the subconscious through to physical body dissolving interior boxes, trunks and cupboards where bad and sad memories fester. Thistle heals old heart wounds helping to melt the armour over your heart due to rejection in companionship. It protects you from giving your heart to manipulative people or dubious beliefs, and fighting or struggling for love. Complementary therapists have long believed that fat or excessive weight is a form of protection, and I believe that this essence may help in weight reduction.

Pipil Tzin-Tzintli *(Salvia divinorum)*
LEADER

Alternative names: Diviner's Sage, Herb of the Shepherdess, Herb of the Virgin
Country: Mexico
Recommended source: Sovereignty Essences
Combined essence: Spring Equinox Goddess by Sovereignty Essences

In Essence

A rare sage that grows in the hidden ravines of Oaxaca, Mexico, and was used by the Mazatec Indians

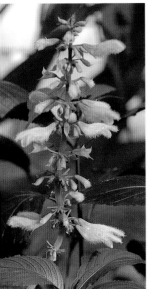

for ritual divinations, Pipil Tzin-Tzintli has that extraordinary exhilarating aroma, which is released when you stroke the leaf. As a flower essence it recognizes and works with your vibrational energy systems and has been found to be particularly beneficial in aiding psychic awareness, meditation, clairvoyance, divination, visions, and contacting higher beings. Pipil Tzin-Tzintli essence makes the intangible tangible. It allows the flexibility of understanding, the multiplicity of creation – and yet the mind is calmed and peaceful.

Jasmine – White *(Jasminum officinale)*
HELPER

Country: India, Persia, Europe
Recommended source: Gaia Essences
Combined essence: Mary – Purification by Gaia Essences

In Essence

The queen of flowers, Jasmine is famed for its fragrant white blooms and sweet aroma; Borneo women roll Jasmine blossoms in their oiled hair before bed. Energetically, it's about self-love and is ideal for those who have lost sight of the loveable person they are. Feelings of unworthiness and loneliness can be a huge burden and make you feel totally exhausted. Move forward: if you are in a stagnant puddle get out – it really is better on dry land.

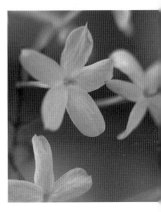

Casuarina Flowers *(Casuarina equisetifolia)*
LEADER, HELPER & MIMICKER

Alternative name: Horsetail She-Oak (flowers)
Country: Australia, Malaysia
Recommended source: Bodylink Essences

In Essence

The bright red, dainty little flowers of the Casuarina could have been leaves but decided to sprout as flowers instead, so they represent freedom from tribal energy – just like the flower essence. Use this cleansing essence to stand out from the crowd in a positive way and show the way forward. With more life force you have life, weather the storms better, are flexible and are unstoppable.

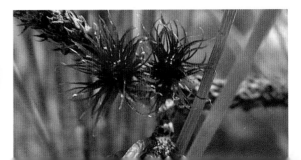

Orange – Citrus (*Citrus sinensis*)
LEADER

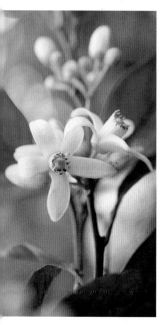

Alternative names: Bigarade Orange, Bigaradier, Bitter Orange, China Orange, Seville Orange, (Sweet) Portugal Orange
Country: India, China, Spain, Madeira
Recommended source: Sabian Essences

In Essence

The white, curled and intensely scented flowers of the Orange produce neroli essential oil (an ingredient of eau de cologne) and the fruit's peel is made into a bitter Orange oil that is an uplifting and energizing tonic. Cleansing and revitalizing, Orange Citrus essence reinforces the energy field, so that the body's immunity can reclaim its power and work more effectively. It deals with creative vitality and increases sexual power. Gradually, by cleansing and clearing the body of negativity surrounding your own sexuality, you can resolve established issues of social conditioning, guilt, insecurity and abuse. The essence can also be helpful for healing scar tissue.

Venus Orchid (*Anguloa clowesii*)
HELPER

Alternative names: Crib of Venus, Tulip Orchid
Country: Colombia, Peru
Recommended source: Korte Essences

In Essence

Found high in the hills and mountains of South America, this magnificent flower takes a long time to mature, but when it does it has an exquisite fragrance that is used in perfumery. Venus Orchid essence is the archetypal feminine essence. It stimulates the yin,

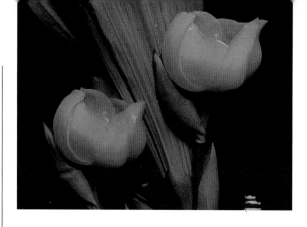

helping to nurture qualities within you such as attentive listening, understanding, gentleness and love. Use this essence for all levels of the physical body, helping to relax a stressed back of head, neck and jaw area.

Clay – Cornish
HELPER & MIMICKER

Country: England
Recommended source: Gaia Essences

In Essence

Traditionally Clay is used as a cleanser, both externally for the skin and internally for the intestines. Cornish Clay essence helps to increase the body's receptiveness to healing. It represents toxin release and total mind and body cleansing, and will balance the intestinal tract flora, cell salts, lymphatics, thymus and pineal gland, helping to resolve skin problems, allergies, ear or eye problems, shingles and sciatica, and encourage tissue regeneration.

Frangipani (*Plumeria*)
HELPER

Alternative names: Dead Man's Fingers, Pua Melia, Temple Tree
Country: America (Hawaii)
Recommended source: Gaia Essences

In Essence

White, yellow, pink, red, or pastel in colour, Frangipani flowers are often used to decorate temples. In Nature it represents 'nurture' and as an essence it allows healing energy to enter all levels of the energy body. This most beautiful flower mothers you, and should remind you to nurture your inner child and cherish your unique identity. When you feel sad or alone, rub some of this essence on your solar plexus, forehead and wrists for subtle comfort. Add it to body lotions, baths or atomizers to nurture your inner being. A popular flower in perfumery, this essence is particular helpful for those people who dislike themselves or put everyone else's welfare first and have no energy left for their own well-being.

Plum (*Prunus domestica*)
HELPER

Alternative name: Prune
Country: Asia, Europe
Recommended source: Sovereignty Essences
Combined essence: Beltane Goddess by Sovereignty Essences

In Essence

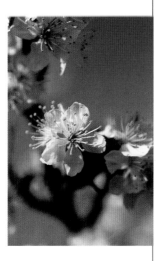

Plum is a small tree popular for its pretty flowers, which appear before the leaves. Cultivated as far back as Roman times, the spiky thorns of the wild tree have long been lost. Medicinally, prunes (dried Plums) are mildly laxative and rich in iron, and stewed prunes make a nourishing diet when you're feeling poorly. Plum essence helps to increase self-motivation and self-worth. It gives a practical solution to problems, and helps the highest spiritual energy enter into the material world; an increase in awareness of your surroundings leads to a more effective use of personal power. Think of it as having a good clear-out – when you are constipated, physically as well as mentally you feel sluggish and full of junk, but when that's cleared you are more comfortable with and aware of the world about you, not worrying about who you are inside yourself.

Aaron's Rod (*Verbascum thapsus*)
LEADER

Alternative names: Adam's Flannel, Beggar's Stalk, Blanket Herb, Clown's Lungwort, Common Mullein, Fluffweed, Golden Rod, Hag's Taper, Jacob's Staff, Jupiter's Staff, Old Man's Flannel, Our Lady's Flannel, Rag Paper, Shepherd's Staff, Velvet Dock, Velvet Plant, Woollen
Country: Britain, Europe, Asia, North America
Recommended source: Rising Serpent Essences

In Essence

The name Aaron's Rod comes from this plant's appearance – one solitary, stout, upright stem. The leaves, flowers and stem have tiny hairs that irritate the throat of animals or humans, so the plant is generally left alone to grow wild and free. Much superstition surrounds this plant: Ulysses chose it to protect himself against the wiles of Circe, in India it is still considered a safeguard against magic and evil spirits, and names such as 'Hag's Taper' are linked to the superstition that witches used it to make lamps and candles. Medicinally, due to its astringent, emollient and antispasmodic properties, Aaron's Rod has been used to treat the lungs, chest and bowels. The whole plant seems to possess slightly sedative and narcotic properties. Aaron's Rod essence works at the throat chakra in the spiritual layer of the physical body and works its way through to the leads of the spiritual body. It's ideal when you need the courage and conviction to follow your spiritual path, and for those who tend to doubt their intuition and ignore their 'gut' instincts.

Heartsease (*Viola tricolor*)
HELPER

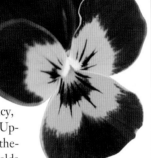

Alternative names:
(*Anglo-Saxon*)
Banewort,
Banwort, Bird's
Eye, Bullweed,
Call-Me-to-You,
Cuddle Me, Cull Me,
Godfathers and
Godmothers, Herb Constancy,
Herb Trinitatis, Jack-Jump-Up-
and-Kiss-Me, Kiss-Her-in-the-
Buttery, Kit-Run-in-the-Fields,
Live-in-Idleness, Love Idol, Love-in-
Idleness, Love-Lies-Bleeding, Loving Idol, Meet-Me-in-
the-Entry, (*French*) Pensée, Pink-Eyed-John, Pink-o'-
the-Eye, Stepmother, Three-Faces-under-a-Hood,
Wild Pansy
Country: Worldwide
Recommended source: Ilminster Essences,
Green Man Essences
Combined essences: Winter Solstice by Sovereignty
Essences; Gaia – The Preserver by Gaia Essences

In Essence

Heartsease, or the little Wild Pansy, is a much-loved
garden flower across the globe. Each flower has three to
four colours and, to my mind, looks like a family of
butterflies. A popular medicinal plant in ancient times
for the plague and sickness, Heartsease has anti-
inflammatory, anti-allergenic, antibacterial and anti-
fungal properties; it is popular in natural health products
as it offers a rich source of antioxidant and nutritious
extracts. It is also used in the homoeopathic treatment of
eczema, psoriasis and other skin conditions. Essence of
Heartsease helps to fill energy holes, rather like the way
it grows in a garden wall. It is very healing and helps
repair damage to the aura, especially from long-standing
emotional hurts. Heartsease also helps to fight off
unwanted external energy, thereby increasing intuition
and boosting your ability to focus. Use the essence for
problems in relationships, where you have built walls
and become thick-skinned or find it hard to open your
heart for fear of being hurt.

Marsh Helleborine (*Epipactis palustris*)
HELPER

Country: Europe, Asia, Ireland, Japan
Recommended source: Silvercord Essences

In Essence

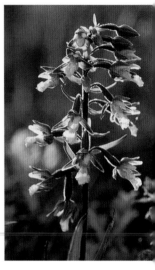

Now rather scarce, Marsh
Helleborine is a creeping plant of
low, marshy ground. The amount
of energy available from Marsh
Helleborine essence gives a
feeling of really being looked
after; feeling safe, it is easy to let
go. The affirmation is: 'I am at
peace.' This essence also works by
enhancing the soul body to
overcome negativity and disperse
blockages in the astral body. As
an essence Marsh Helleborine
enhances the soul level, in either
a place or person, clearing out
negative energies and producing
feelings of tranquillity and
harmony. Another use is to disperse blockages in the
psyche of those who have become withdrawn as a result
of a trauma such as grief.

Hellebore (*Helleborus viridis*)
HELPER

Alternative name: Green Hellebore
Country: Britain, Southern Europe
Recommended source: Gaia Essences
Combined essence: Demeter – Hope by Gaia Essences

In Essence

Increasingly popular in damp, shady gardens,
Hellebore is easy to grow and has attractive winter
flowers and foliage. The root has many medicinal
properties: it is cardiac, diuretic, emetic, irritant,
violently narcotic and a drastic purgative and is
recommended for those with high blood pressure. It is
also good for the heart and to bring on menstrual flow

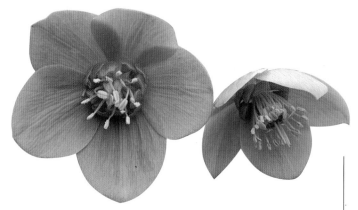

and expel parasitic worms. Hellebore essence is more about growing old gracefully. It helps you to bow down to the passing of time, whether that is getting older or accepting change over a long period of time. I think it's perfect for grumpy old men and women – if they could ever see that they needed anything, of course!

Tulasi *(Ocimum sanctum)*
HELPER

Alternative names: Holy Basil, Tulsi
Country: India
Recommended source: Soul Quintessence System
Combined essence: Christ Ray

In Essence

Native to India and popular in Ayurvedic medicine, Tulasi is greatly revered as a medicine in ancient Indian scriptures and is referred to throughout 5,000 years of written history in the *Vedas*, the oldest texts known to man. No offering to the gods in temple life would be complete without the inclusion of Tulasi. In many homes there were special altars on the veranda where a pot of the herb was kept; every morning and evening the family would perform a ritual prayer to the plant, called 'the protector of life'. Upon someone's death, a leaf from the Tulasi was placed on the breast to facilitate passage to paradise. Medicinally, the herb has

a dizzying array of benefits, being antispasmodic, antidepressant, antiseptic, stimulating and antibacterial, as well as encouraging perspiration and bringing down a fever. It is everything from a general tonic to an appetizer and makes a great insect repellent. Myths and legends about Tulasi say it is used in love potions and 'causes sympathy between human beings'. Beads made from Tulasi are always worn by mystics and yogis to dispel and clean away negative influences. Tulasi essence relates to your birth – past, present and future – on a karmic level. It offers deep healing and realignment, enabling the release of guilt and the sins of old.

Couch Grass – Common
(Elytrigia repens) HELPER

Alternative names: Dog-Grass, Scotch Quelch, Quick-Grass, Twitch-Grass
Country: Britain, Europe, Asia, Australia, North and South America
Recommended source: Silvercord Essences

In Essence

Deeply unpopular with farmers because of its creeping root system Couch Grass is almost impossible to remove once it is established in the soil. Couch Grass root was a popular drink to purify the blood in ancient times and is still taken as a *tisane* in France – it is known to help with cystitis, gout and rheumatism. I highly recommend Couch Grass essence when you need help to slow down, take things easy and recover because it swiftly reduces energy flowing through the valves. Working on the heart chakra by cleansing energy strands, it may help the symptoms of bronchial catarrh, arthritis, rheumatism, cystitis and skin disorders. It is recommended to help you take steps forward and for workaholics.

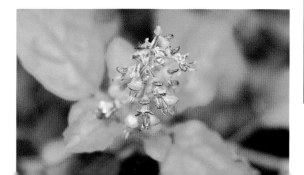

Victorian Christmas Bush
(Prostanthera lasianthos) LEADER

Alternative name: Mint Bush
Country: Australia (east coast)
Recommended source: Sabian Essences

In Essence

With oval-shaped leaves surrounded by sprays of white, pink, or mauve blossoms, the Victorian Christmas bush grows by creeks and in the moist shade of dense, wet forests. When not in flower, a menthol fragrance emanates from the plant when brushed. Essence-wise,

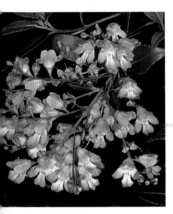

if you feel as if the lights are on but no one is home, take a break and this essence will re-boot your energy field. If you've pressed the enter button too many times, this essence re-boots your system and says, 'Hey, it's not so bad after all.' Once all programs are running as they should, insecurity ebbs; you feel protected, nurtured, serene and in harmony.

Tears of Christ (water from the waterfall, Geiranger Fjord) LEADER

Alternative names: (Norwegian) Geirangerfjorden
Country: Norway (Geiranger Fjord)
Recommended source: Bodylink Essences

In Essence

One of Mother Nature's masterpieces, Geiranger is often called 'the most beautiful fjord in the world', and this is no exaggeration – the landscape will leave you breathless. If you love wandering through beautiful scenery, many walks let you enjoy the peace and quiet and impressive natural beauty at your leisure. Tears of Christ essence maintains that the cliffs that rise from the fjord are a masterpiece of split personality. There are faces, animals, birds – just about everything

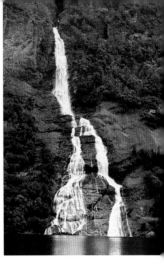

imaginable – to be seen in the undulating and craggy rocks. This particular 'face' looked very much like pictures of Christ and the waterfalls appeared to come from the eyes, so I couldn't resist this name when I made the essence. Fed up with being made the scapegoat for other people's failures? Always feel like you're being deceived and misled? This essence offers protection from evil and it will make you feel less vulnerable. Often when you badly want something, you compromise yourself to achieve it and this can leave you open to abuse and deception – especially in business and money matters. Tears of Christ essence helps you to stop and ask what really is important. Injustice, anger and martyrdom become a thing of the past.

Rose She-Oak (*Allocasuarina torulosa*) LEADER

Alternative name: Forest Oak
Country: Australia (Queensland, New South Wales)
Recommended source: Sabian Essences

In Essence

Rose She-Oak is a rare, exotic timber often used in wood turnings and for knife handles; the grain of the wood is a reddish pinky-brown, with a rose-like scent. In essence, Rose She-Oak is a leader and is great for times when the heart has received a direct shock. It represents 'wholeness' and works at a core/membrane level to increase the take-up of power directly to the heart. Ideal for anyone who finds they have no willpower, or suffers from lack of interest, feeling weak, procrastinating and out of sync with their inner self, this essence helps you recognise your attributes, and promotes inner wisdom and power.

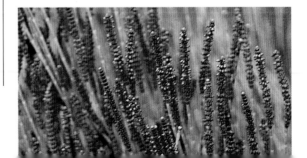

Red River Gum

(*Eucalyptus camaldulensis*) LEADER

Alternative name: Euc rostratus
Country: Australia
Recommended source: Sabian Essences

In Essence

Red River Gum is a common and widespread tree along the streams and rivers of much of mainland Australia. The tree itself can reach 1,000 years old, and Aboriginals have long used the wood for canoes. The way it grows in heavy clay means that it is often used on flood plains to stabilize the ground – and herein lies the link, because we often feel 'bogged down' ourselves, as if our feet were in clay. This essence has the ability to help you lighten up and rise above boggy conditions. In essence, Red River Gum helps to expand your internal energy to new levels. Perfect for those times when you feel fearful, isolated or weighed down, it helps to restore the lightness, humour and wisdom to rise above it all – but still remain grounded – giving you the strength to like yourself as you are.

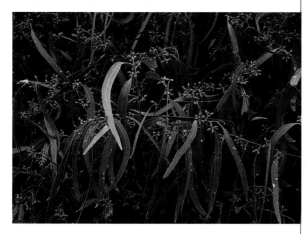

Silver Princess (*Eucalyptus caesia*)
LEADER

Alternative name: Gungurru
Country: Western Australia
Recommended source: Bodylink Essences

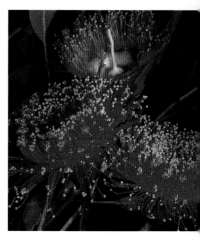

In Essence

Unlike the typical image of a eucalyptus, Silver Princess is a much smaller tree with beautiful pinky-red flowers that are fine and fluffy with a dramatic 'pointy' yellow centre. Energetically Silver Princess helps with creative direction and in finding the purpose in your life. The essence has a direct link with the reasoning of the body – working directly on the second chakra, which can be helpful with finding your life direction. The sacral chakra addresses issues of self-esteem and confidence – if these are at their maximum you can follow your inner direction without hindrance.

Centaurea (*Centaurea montana*)
LEADER

Alternative names: Knapweed, Mountain Bluet, Mountain Knapweed, Perennial Bachelor's Buttons, Perennial Cornflower
Country: Europe
Recommended source: Bodylink Essences

In Essence

With brilliant blue to pale mauve blossoms like ripped tissue paper, Centaurea is one of the most striking wildflowers. The flowers have stimulating properties and provoke menstrual flow, and are also an active ingredient in eye care products, such as treatments for conjunctivitis and eye make-up remover. Energetically, Centaurea means opening your eyes to reality. Disbelief follows shock, leaving you unable to recover from a situation too painful to deal with – and you may tell yourself stories to help the situation become bearable. Centaurea essence allows you to deal with the truth, flipping energy from negative to positive.

Green Alkanet
(Pentaglottis sempervirens) LEADER

Alternative name: Evergreen Bugloss
Country: Britain
Recommended source: Rising Serpent Essences

In Essence

A member of the borage family, this rough, hairy plant grows in the hedgerows, in damp, shady woods, and along the banks and grassy verges. Green Alkanet works like a weed, starting at the heart chakra of the mental level and working right through the core to the spiritual matrix and energy valves. This grounding essence is ideal for a person irritable about dealing

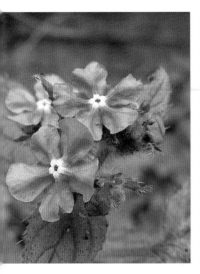

with practicalities – someone who may be intelligent, but lacks common sense. This state of mind is often due to trauma (especially from fire) in other lives so the soul feels unsafe in the body, creating a sense of not wanting to participate fully, which manifests as spiritual snobbery. Use this essence to help with allergies of an unknown source, and problems with heat or burns.

Silverband (water from the Silverband Falls, Gariwerd, Grampians National Park) LEADER

Country: Australia (Victoria)
Recommended source: Bodylink Essences

In Essence

An oasis of natural fauna and flora, the Grampians National Park outside Melbourne in Australia is home to the Silverband Falls, an extraordinary 20-metre high waterfall. There is an eerie, almost surreal feeling when

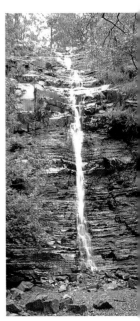

you stand facing the water – there is silence, not a splash, nothing: just a wonderful, peaceful ambience that touches everyone who visits this little-known fall. This is because the water does not fall into a pool, but disappears underground and re-emerges further downstream. The beauty of waterfalls – along with other invigorating environments in Nature, such as mountain tops and beaches – is that the air circulating in these magical places is said to contain tens of thousands of negative oxygen ions (a good thing I assure you), creating lighter, clearer air around you and lightening the spirits at the same time. In an essence, Silverband helps to bring hidden emotions up from the subconscious to the surface. Energetically, it accesses the subconscious and allows your emotions to float to the surface to be dealt with easily.

Timothy Grass *(Phleum pratense)*
HELPER & MIMICKER

Alternative name: Timothy
Country: Britain
Recommended source: Silvercord Essences

In Essence

A common meadow grass, Timothy Grass is probably most familiar as pet feed for rabbits and guinea pigs, although extracts of the plant have recently been found to help arrest certain cancers and tumour growths (including sarcomas). As a plant essence, Timothy Grass works on the heart chakra and is the perfect remedy for helping you to love yourself and to enable you to love others. It is especially useful for healing the intestines, stomach and bowels.

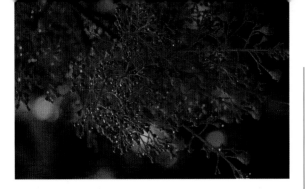

Flame Tree (*Brachychiton acerifolius*)
LEADER

Alternative name: Illawarra Flame Tree
Country: Australia
Recommended source: Sabian Essences

In Essence

The Flame Tree is one of the world's most beautiful flowering trees – the small flowers are produced by the thousand, making the entire tree appear flame-red. The tree grows fast and tall and loves the sun; similarly, its essence is about strength, courage and the ability to manifest goals, yet stay grounded. It inspires structure. Ideal for those times when you feel timid, insecure, unfocused and unsure of yourself, this essence allows the body to listen to the soul, connecting through the chakras to a higher wisdom and self-knowledge.

Silver Banksia (*Banksia marginata*)
LEADER

Country: Australia (New South Wales, Queensland, Victoria)
Recommended source: Sabian Essences

In Essence

Usually found in the typical Australian forests of hard-leaved plants that stretch from the coast to mountainous areas, Silver Banksia has fluffy rounded flower spikes. This adaptable plant can grow in even the poorest soils, but must see the sunshine. The flowers are filled with a sweet nectar, which can be sucked directly or washed out with water to make a refreshing beverage. Silver Banksia essence is perfect for those who dwell on past hurt, pain and blame, are in constant fear, have some blocked

trauma, and are generally stuck in a negative outlook. Energetically, it helps to heighten an awareness to the core of the major energy lines. The physical feels more grounded and able to cope, as if there is an army on your side, and allows you to develop a fresh outlook and to let go of negativity, encouraging inner growth and much more positive achievements.

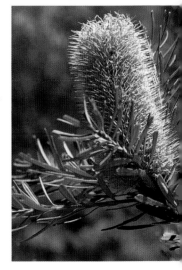

Lime – Linden (*Tilia x europaea*) LEADER

Alternative names: Common Lime, Flores Tiliae, Linden Flowers, Linn Flowers, Tilia cordata, Tilia intermedia, Tilia platyphyllos, Tilia vulgaris, Tilleul
Country: Europe
Recommended source: Green Man Essences

In Essence

The honey from the Lime's yellowish-white flowers is regarded as the best in the world, and is used exclusively in medicine and in liqueurs. The wood is valuable for carving and making furniture. Linden tea is still used on the Continent, especially in France, where stores of dried Lime flowers are kept for making 'Tilleul', as a household remedy for indigestion and nerves. Lime essence helps to decrease an oversensitive cross energy, allowing the body to focus on a spiritual endeavour. It is useful for when you want to shift levels of

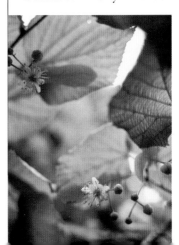

consciousness without disorientation, helping to lessen past behaviour programming, erase doubts and fears, and calm the anxiety related to the practical use of your psychic and healing potential.

African Violet (*Saintpaulia*)
HELPER

Country: Kenya, South Africa
Recommended source: Gaia Essences
Combined essence: Hathor – The Flame by Gaia Essences

In Essence

Growing high in the rocky mountains of Kenya, every aspect of the African Violet, from its purple colour (the seventh chakra is purple and represents spiritual enlightenment) to its tiny golden stamens (like the sun and its golden rays of wisdom), reflects its spirituality. Signifying true enlightenment, African Violets are a sign of rejuvenation, internal cleansing and spiritual release. The essence makes connections and transcends boundaries, helping to balance the nervous system and create harmony within the mental and physical body. I also love to use this essence mixed with Watermelon and Ginger essences for skin rejuvenation.

White Mangrove (*Laguncularia racemosa*)
LEADER

Alternative name: Mangle Blanco
Country: Australia
Recommended source: Sabian Essences

In Essence

This flowering tree grows beside freshwater creeks, billabongs and swamps in the Northern Territory of Australia and can be recognized by the two bumps (glands) on its round, leathery, slightly fleshy leaves. The flowers bloom in

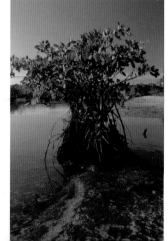

small spikes and it has grooved, almond-shaped fruits. Reported to be astringent and a tonic, White Mangrove is a folk remedy for dysentery. The healing quality of the essence is to release and heal mental prejudice, allowing the heart to open without prejudgement. Often the seeds of this prejudice have been sown for a long time – in many cases it is generational, as in countries where religious prejudice is passed on and accepted by the young without question. Many prejudices develop because of cultural belief that nothing can be done. This essence has the potential to allow you to fully experience and be open to new shifts in perception and all the associated changes, on both a head and a heart level. It promotes openness to new experiences and people, and healthy questioning of traditional standards and beliefs. For times when you feel tearful and highly strung and are suppressing your emotions, this essence will make you more intuitive, caring, balanced and put in touch with your feelings.

Cyclamen (*Hederifolium*)
HELPER

Alternative name: Hardy Cyclamen
Country: Europe (France, through Italy, Corsica, Sardinia, Sicily, Croatia, Bosnia, Serbia, Albania, Bulgaria, Greece)
Recommended source: Gaia Essences
Combined essence: Athena – The Warrior by Gaia Essences

In Essence

Cyclamen inhabits woodland, scrubs and rocky hillsides, often in shady areas rather than full sun. Each delicate pink flower nods downward at the end of a slender stem and there is a purple-magenta V-shaped blotch at the base of each petal. In essence, Cyclamen helps to release deep-seated trauma in the second sacral chakra. Long established, harboured grudges can be released and you will find that you grow towards forgiveness and positivity.

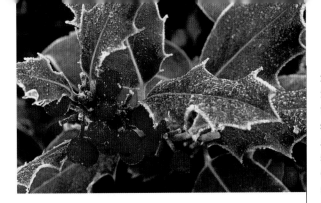

Holly (*Ilex aquifolium*)
HELPER

Alternative names: Christ's Thorn, Holm, Holme Chase, Holy Tree, Hulm, Hulver Bush
Country: Central and Southern Europe
Recommended source: Bodylink, Green Man, Sovereignty Essences, Bach Collection by Sun Essences
Combined essences: Heart to Heart by Bodylink Essences; Winter Solstice by Sovereignty Essences

In Essence

Holly, one of the most striking trees in the wintry woodland, is linked to Christmas in our hearts and minds – Yuletide decorations derived from a Roman custom of sending boughs to friends during the Saturnalia festival. Every part of the plant has a stimulating medicinal use for ailments such as catarrh, pleurisy, smallpox, fever and rheumatism. Holly essence is particularly effective in times of emotional distress, panic, agitation, misery and loneliness. Taking the essence is an active expression of self-love. It balances and restores inner control creating a sense of balance and positive energy. Goodwill to mankind – every single day of the year.

Golden Wattle (*Acacia pycnantha*)
LEADER

Alternative name: Wattle Bark
Country: Australia
Recommended source: Sabian Essences

In Essence

With its adorable yellow-gold pompom flowers, the Golden Wattle has long been regarded as Australia's

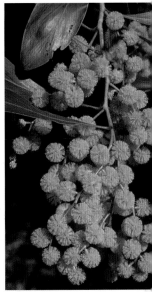

national flower. Its pollen-rich flowers emit a sweet, oily gum that can be sucked like candy or soaked in water to make a jelly. As a plant, Golden Wattle has amazing powers of regeneration (especially after a bush fire); as an essence it also represents growth and can turn a negative, lazy, detached, apathetic attitude into an energetic, deeply fulfilled, uplifting soul, well connected to the universe. In my experience, subtle hearing is also increased to help you 'listen to your own needs'.

Purple Iris (*Iris germanica*)
HELPER

Alternative name: Bearded Iris
Country: Britain, Europe
Recommended source: Gaia Essences
Combined essence: Hathor – The Flame by Gaia Essences

In Essence

Named after the Greek goddess of the rainbow, Purple Iris grows wild throughout the Northern Hemisphere. The Ancients used it as a perfume and medicine, and the French adopted it as a powerful symbol of the monarchy, the sacred *fleur-de-lis*. In Turkey, graveyards are decorated with this heavenly flower, and in Italy it is an important ingredient – orris – in the perfume industry. Often massed in high Himalayan bogs, clinging to life on an arid Greek hillside, or lining the banks of a nearby canal, Purple Iris embraces its surroundings, wherever they may be. As an essence, it overcomes deep resentment and – just like bad breath or body odour – it's nasty and off-putting to others. But in my mind, with Purple Iris 'stinking thinking' turns into 'happy chappy'.

Blue Gum (*Eucalyptus globulus*)
LEADER & HELPER

Alternative names: Blue Gum Tree, Fever Tree, Stringy Bark Tree
Country: Australia, North and South Africa, India, Southern Europe
Recommended source: Sabian Essences

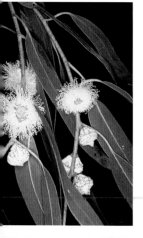

In Essence

The button-like leaves of this towering tree are laden with the active oil eucalyptol, the most powerful antiseptic of its kind – aromatic stimulant, antiseptic gargle and anti-malarial. In veterinary practice, eucalyptus oil is administered to horses with flu, dogs with distemper, and to treat septicaemia in all animals. In the plant world, eucalyptus represents communication. Blue Gum essence promotes clear communication lines between the crown and sacral chakra levels. Regular use ensures communication within the body, turning an uncommunicative, flighty, unsure and 'living in the past' aspect into one with clarity of speech, focus, assurance and understanding.

Citrine
HELPER

Alternative name: Citrine quartz
Country: Brazil
Recommended source: Gaia Essences

In Essence

Citrine is an amber-coloured gemstone, which in ancient times was carried as a protection against evil thoughts and snakebite. It reflects the colour yellow, which is all about optimism and works on the second and third chakras to link to the spiritual seventh chakra. It is ideal for those who harbour negative emotions: of never being good enough; of losing control, being ruled by emotions or quickly shattered by criticism; or lacking focus. Citrine essence is warming, comforting, lifegiving. It brings personal power, focus, endurance, creativity and beginnings.

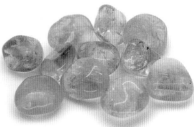

It promotes self-discipline and the ability to make money. It can lighten up the darkest corner of your life, alleviate destructive tendencies, reinforce self-confidence, and bring laughter and cohesion back between family members. Citrine also links to circulation, thyroid, muscle toxins, digestion, and the body's assimilation of vitamins A, C and E.

Silky Oak (*Grevillea robusta*)
LEADER

Country: Australia (New South Wales, Queensland)
Recommended source: Sabian Essences

In Essence

Amid temperate rainforests, this immense, drought-resistant evergreen tree grows incredibly fast. Its leaves are a source of rutin, and its flowers are hermaphrodite (containing both male and female organs) and are one of the richest sources of nectar – it falls in showers when you lightly shake the flowers. As an essence, Silky Oak is all about promoting self-love and self-confidence. It works by allowing the feminine (yin) energy to play its part in connecting you to your intuitive self. It helps to increase your confidence by experiencing a soft approach to disputes, using the qualities of listening, intuition and reasoning rather than to 'fight to win'.

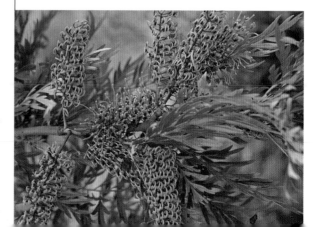

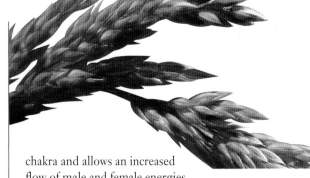

Snow Gum (*Eucalyptus pauciflora*)
LEADER & HELPER

Country: Australia (New South Wales, Victoria)
Recommended source: Sabian Essences

In Essence

A smaller eucalyptus, Snow Gum only grows to around six metres in height, but it's fast and in leaf all year round, with flowers that are loved by bees. Indeed this particular species, with its beautiful, silvery bark, is

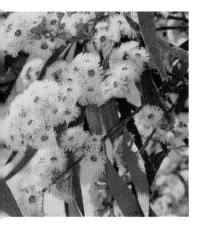

renowned for attracting wildlife. A very knowing tree, Snow Gum works well in an essence as both a leader and a helper and is great for attaining wisdom and knowledge. Energetically it shuts down the physical valve so that the body is infused with expanded spiritual energy. A lovely way to shut out the physical world and learn more about yourself, Snow Gum essence helps us to overcome issues of not feeling worthy, childishness, lack of vision, and 'I can't cope', allowing us to feel better connected to Nature and become a true survivor.

Velvet Bentgrass (*Agrostis canina*)
HELPER

Country: America
Recommended source: Silvercord Essences

In Essence

Velvet Bentgrass has the finest texture of all the bentgrasses and is one of the oldest varieties. It is used for lawns and golf courses in Europe and was brought to the United States to create early putting greens, because of its fine texture and ability to be clipped closely. Velvet Bentgrass essence affects the crown chakra and allows an increased flow of male and female energies, mainly to the throat area, helping to improve your intuition at all levels. If you feel you have become firmly stuck in a rut, it also helps with the decision-making process.

Crocus – Purple (*Crocus*)
HELPER

Alternative names: Crocus, Karcom, Krokos, (*Arabian*) Zaffer
Country: Europe
Recommended source: Gaia Essences
Combined essence: Hathor – The Flame by Gaia Essences

In Essence

Always having a particular place in a gardener's affections, the Crocus is one of the first flowers of the year to bloom, even while there is still snow. Memories of childhood walks in the woods include seeing whole patches of lilac-mauve flowers, gleaming in the sunshine and alive with foraging bees. Their very innocence touches the heart and makes us feel a spark of joy. The Crocus multiplies quickly below ground, even in crevices and cracks in paths – but no one ever considers them invasive because they are so charming and welcome. Crocus essence is the perfect reflection of the flower, helping you to overcome grief, loss and despair, creating a more joyous outlook on life and helping the stress to disappear.

Buddleia (*Buddleia davidii*)
LEADER

Alternative names: Butterfly Bush, Empire Blue, Summer Lilac
Country: China, Britain (Naturalized)
Recommended source: Bodylink Essences
Combined essence: Buddleia Butterfly

In Essence

Buddleia's pretty tubular flowers are rich in nectar and often extremely fragrant. The flower buds are known to be antispasmodic and good for the eyes, and have an action similar to vitamin P, reducing the fragility of blood vessels in the skin and of the small intestine. Buddleia essence represents sweetness and metamorphosis and works on the solar plexus chakra to release the energy band around the upper abdomen. When you are hurt

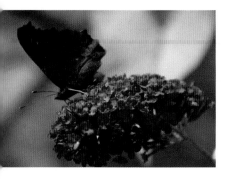

you retreat to recuperate, but if you stay in this state for too long you can become a victim and close your heart to limit the pain; over time, this can result in a tight energy band that links to the diaphragm.

Heartburn, excessive stomach acid and other digestive disturbances can follow. As I made this essence, a peacock butterfly sat on the flower the entire time, symbolizing a higher perspective, helping you come out of hibernation and letting old hurts go, releasing the energy between heart and stomach. Buddleia allows energy to flow around the centre and follow its natural pathway.

Giant Honey Myrtle

(*Melaleuca diosmifolia*) LEADER

Alternative name: Green Honey Myrtle
Country: Australia
Recommended source: Sabian Essences

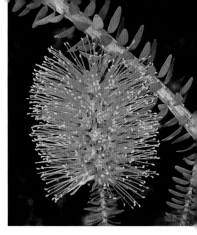

In Essence

The large bottlebrush flower heads of the Giant Honey Myrtle are yellowy green; it has lime-green, crowded, pine-like leaves and forms a large, dense bush. The flowers of this striking shrub are very attractive to birds and it is often planted for hedging. With its small leaves neatly spiralling around the stems, this tenacious plant can cope with pretty much anything thrown at it. When you need increased balance of energy, this essence will halt those feelings of restlessness, of being weighed down, of irritation and make you feel peace, harmony, lightness, assurance and a sense of release.

Sand Rush Grass (*Bulbostylis capillaris*)
HELPER

Alternative names: Hair Sedge, Thread-Leaved Beak-Seed
Country: North and South America (especially California)
Recommended source: Silvercord Essences

In Essence

A deeply resilient hair-like grass that tolerates extreme environmental conditions, Sand Rush Grass is native to California but it is also found in other areas of North America and in South America. When used as an essence, Sand Rush Grass acts as a deep cleanse to the whole system, flushing toxins effectively through the body's own filtering systems. This is a great essence to help skin conditions, the skeletal frame and also rheumatism.

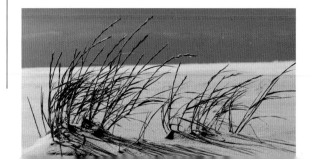

Past Life Orchid
(Paphiopedilum harrysianum) HELPER

Country: Caribbean
Recommended source: Korte Essences

In Essence

Past Life Orchid has long leaves with rounded tips, which grow in the shape of a fan. It has a very ornate, pinky-red flower on a single stalk, but the precious essence is only taken from the buds that have just opened. Past Life Orchid essence helps to connect you with your subconscious, and puts you back into your past, to soothe old sorrows and so improve memory. Energetically it helps to access your soul records; this may help you retrieve knowledge that can resolve present challenges. Ultimately, it helps you explore the depths of your being and subconscious, to find answers to the everyday and deeper questions of life.

Grounding Opuntia Cactus
(Opuntia dejecta) HELPER & MIMICKER

Alternative names: Spiny Nopal
Country: Cuba, Central America
Recommended source: Korte Essences

In Essence

Grounding Opuntia Cactus is a typical low-growing cactus, sturdy and resilient in the extreme heat of the sun. In essence, it activates the first base chakra, connecting you more strongly with the Earth. Increased cross energy or energetic force field at the hips gives more protection to the base chakra and lower extremities. Taking this essence gives greater stability, helping you to experience inner peace and better self-awareness.

Heather *(Calluna vulgaris)*
HELPER

Country: Britain, Northern Europe
Recommended source: Soul Quintessence System, Bach Collection by Sun Essences

In Essence

A rare flower seen amidst Britain's desolate moors and highlands, Heather often appears out of place in these locations, yet our hearts are always glad for its presence. In essence, Heather allows a soul–heart connection. It helps maintain a sense of purity and simplicity in the heart and promotes inner exploration, contemplation and reflection as a natural opening for simple discernment. This will assist in decision-making and helps you recognize when you are suppressing your first feelings or intuition and not trusting in your guidance on 'the heart of the matter'. The key is to maintain equilibrium through simplicity. To maintain simplicity is an art you must apply in order to grow and learn in a healthy, progressive fashion because we all tend to complicate our lives and divert ourselves from the real task at hand. Complications quickly build up when the spirit can no longer guide you in your day-to-day dealings; you then resort to quick-fix solutions. You don't have to do what others want just to keep the peace, or avoid dealing with issues. You need to be able to say what you really feel and to express your needs as they arise. Being unable to get things off your chest can result in more confusion, more stress and more anxiety, triggering sudden outbursts. Heather essence can be used to align imbalances of the breath – chest (heart, breasts, lungs), circulation, skin, hair and nails. This essence is also great for space clearing and meditation, because it creates a peaceful ambience. It is perfect when dealing with dysfunctional personal, family or community issues.

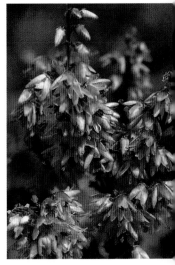

Iolite

LEADER, HELPER & MIMICKER

Alternative names: Gem of the Vikings, Shaman's Strength, Water Sapphire
Country: India, Sri Lanka, Mozambique, Zimbabwe, Brazil
Recommended source: Gaia Essences

In Essence

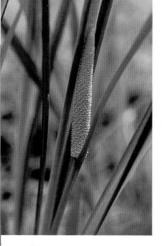

Iolite comes from the Greek *ios*, which means violet. Iolite is usually a purplish-blue when it is cut properly; the richer the blue, the better the stone. Viking mariners used thin pieces as the world's first polarizing filter – looking through an Iolite lens, they could determine the exact position of the sun and navigate safely to new lands and back. A good stone for helping you to find direction in life, Iolite helps open the pathway for the spiritual. It connects the throat, brow and crown chakras to open a subtle and gentle connection with your higher self, which may manifest as sudden bursts of intuition, along with a higher awareness for guidance or purpose. Iolite essence also helps you to release discord and protects from negative energies. Great in the workplace, it can help you to feel comfortable as a leader and make others accept you in that role more easily. This essence will prevent you from allowing others to walk all over you, allowing your emotions to control you, or making a martyr of yourself. It is a good healing stone.

Sweet Flag Grass (*Acorus calamus*)

HELPER

Alternative names: Cinnamon Sedge, Gladdon, Myrtle Grass, Myrtle Sedge, Sweet Cane, Sweet Myrtle, Sweet Root, Sweet Rush, Sweet Sedge
Country: Britain, Europe, Asia, North America
Recommended source: Silvercord Essences

In Essence

Sweet Flag Grass is a vigorous, reed-like, aquatic plant that flourishes in ditches, lakes, streams and marshy places. Often confused with an Iris, it has erect, sword-shaped leaves and a pleasant odour, and until quite recently was freely strewn on the floors of churches at festivals and often in private houses. Sweet Flag Grass has a very long history of medicinal use in many herbal traditions. It is widely used in modern herbal medicine as an aromatic stimulant and mild tonic. In Ayurvedic medicine it is highly valued as a rejuvenator for the brain and nervous system and as a remedy for digestive disorders, and a homoeopathic remedy is made from the roots for the treatment of flatulence, dyspepsia, anorexia and gall bladder problems. Take Sweet Flag Grass flower essence to bring you strength for new beginnings. It affects the brow and the heart and helps to unravel cross energies that cause a build-up above the throat and the abdomen.

Maize (*Zea mays*)

HELPER

Alternative names: Indian Corn, Sweet Corn
Country: North and South America, Caribbean
Recommended source: Silvercord Essences

In Essence

Maize is a yellow cereal that grows in abundance in the United States and is hugely popular with Americans, for making hominy, samp and a porridge called 'mush'. A diuretic and a mild stimulant, Maize is easily digested by the human body. Corn bread, made from Maize, is nourishing and suitable for those suffering from kidney or liver diseases. Mexicans make 'chikka' from fermented Maize, a drink that resembles cider. Medically, cornmeal makes a nutritious gruel and is an excellent diet for convalescents; it can also dispel nausea and vomiting in

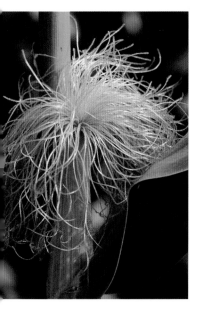

many diseases. Maize makes a good soothing poultice for ulcers, swellings and rheumatic pains, while as an essence it increases energy at the higher crown and spiritual chakras. It works well as a diuretic as it also affects the kidney and bladder, and can be used for arthritis and rheumatism. Use Maize essence to ease the mental process through the solar plexus and to unwind hard, established thought patterns.

Horsetail She-Oak

(Casuarina equisetifolia) LEADER

Alternative names: Australian Pine, Beefwood, Ironwood
Country: Malaysia, Southern Asia, Oceania, Australia, Caribbean
Recommended source: Bodylink Essences

In Essence

Horsetail She-Oak, with its soft, wispy, pine-like branches, is capable of year-round flowering. It grows well in any area, but it's a sun worshipper and prefers the beach: sandy, shell or rocky. The Horsetail She-Oak also grows in sand dunes and sand bars. The wood is popular for boat-building, fences and oars because it is strong, heavy and salt resistant. In folk medicine, Horsetail She-Oak has been used as a tonic, diuretic, and laxative. Energetically, the essence is great for

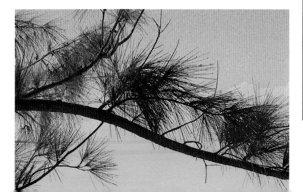

sweeping away the debris that stops you being who you should be: 'Dare to be different', it says, 'Be a leader'. I use this day-in, day-out in the clinic, between clients, to cleanse the space of the issues they leave behind.

Water Moss

(Sphagnum palustre ssp) HELPER

Alternative name: Peat Bog
Country: China, Bhutan, Nepal, India, Thailand
Recommended source: Soul Quintessence System

In Essence

Found mostly near heather, mountains and moors, Water Moss clumps together to form large cushions on the ground. Medically it was once used to heal wounds by helping them knit together. In essence, Water Moss helps when you are avoiding intimacy – appearing open and able to give, but only on a material and superficial level. The symptoms may manifest as intolerance towards others or appearing superior or aloof. Extreme cases may manifest as phobias, inertia or reclusive behaviour – concealing weaknesses rather than confronting, revealing and healing them. When we recognize our weaknesses and strengths regarding intimacy, avoidance and vulnerability, and accept them equally, we begin relating to others with trust. Feeling supported and safe, we release neediness and lack from relationships. Water

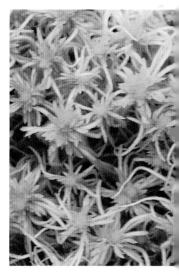

Moss lets you learn to exist for yourself, moving from survival as a way of being; it's all about communication. Throat, ears, thyroid, mouth, teeth, gums and neck problems may all be eased and it also helps release phobias, introversion, an elitist mentality, and grief over separation. Realignment with this essence means reaching for the stars, uniting in spiritual goals, a true feeling of belonging and an absolute sense of connection.

Black Wattle (*Acacia mearnsii*)
LEADER

Alternative name: Gomboom
Country: Australia (Queensland, New South Wales, Tasmania)
Recommended source: Sabian Essences

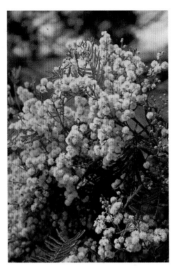

In Essence

A hardy tree that's used in the tanning of soft leather and for paper, the Black Wattle is tolerant of drought, frost and poor soil. Some regard it as an attractive ornamental plant, while others call it the 'green cancer' for the resolute way it spreads vigorously like a weed. In folk medicine, Black Wattle is often used as a styptic or astringent. Working directly on the throat chakra, I find its essence boosts all communication lines between this chakra and the physical body. It relates to trust and works to counteract all negative attitudes such as mistrust, criticism, and self-denial, leaving you to experience only comfort, trust, acknowledgement, openness and self-acceptance.

Birch (*Betula pubescens*)
LEADER

Alternative name: Downy Birch
Country: Britain, Ireland, Europe, Siberia, Central Asia
Recommended source: Soul Quintessence System

In Essence

The Birch bark is anti-inflammatory and has long been used as an astringent for skin conditions such as eczema and psoriasis. The leaves can be used to treat conditions such as gout, rheumatism and kidney stones, and the sweet sap is a diuretic. Birch essence helps you to recognize and reassess your identity. We commonly accept certain characteristics as being part of us; we become over-attached to possessions or status as if they determine our fate, such as: 'I am successful because I am a businessman'; or 'I am useless because I am poor'. This attitude encourages narcissism or defeatism, which may manifest as bodily aversions or resistance to physical incarnations – such as trauma at birth, or childlike body features and characteristics in adults. Your body is an instrument for catalytic change within and without and teaches you to appreciate, transform and transcend matter. Birch helps you understand and respect the divine relationship between body and spirit, so your real quest for identity as a soul can be fulfilled. Also use Birch for skin problems, poor memory and headaches caused by digestive problems.

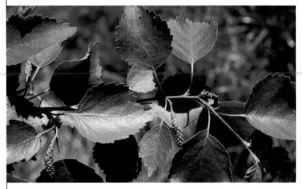

Wavy Hair Grass (*Deschampsia flexuosa*)
HELPER

Country: Britain
Recommended source: Silvercord Essences

In Essence

On wild moors and hills, among the grass, heather and rocks, you may find a bank of Wavy Hair Grass nestling on a dry slope. The delicate, branching stems holding the seed heads are crimped just like wavy hair; the glossy leaves also look a bit like long hairs – and unusually for a grass they are cylindrical, allowing for plenty of moisture retention in the plant's dry, open habitat. A beautiful grass, it blows gently in the breeze

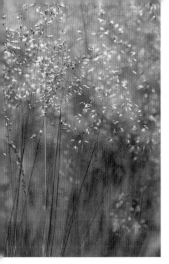

like a full head of hair being lightly tossed around. Great for mind and body metabolism, Wavy Hair Grass essence acts like a tonic – especially for scalp conditions. The physical valve becomes flushed, clearing bodily toxins and giving you an increased awareness. It is a wonderful essence for those who run with the pack and need to step back.

Apple (*Malus domestica*)
LEADER

Country: Northern Hemisphere
Recommended source: Green Man Essences, Bach Collection by Sun Essences

In Essence

An Apple a day keeps the doctor away. Well, this old saying has real meaning if you study the historical virtues of this much-loved fruit. The taste for Apples is one of the earliest and most natural of inclinations; the aroma of Apple pie is a key ingredient in modern perfumery. Rich in vitamins, the Apple is classed as one of the most valuable of the fruits used for relieving scurvy. Popular instinct long ago led to the association of applesauce with rich foods such as pork and goose; the English fancy for eating cheese with Apple pie – an obsolete taste, nowadays – is another example of instinctive inclination. The main value of Apples lies in the malic and tartaric acids that make the fruit and other foods digestible. Ripe, juicy, sour Apples eaten at bedtime will cure some of the worst forms of constipation and even insomnia. As an essence, Apple is detoxifying; it helps to eliminate toxins on all levels and brings in spiritual energies. It cleanses cross energies, balancing the sacral, heart and throat chakras, to release

tension – physical and emotional – clear the mind, ease the breath and even sharpen your hearing. Trust Apple to transform negative emotions.

Rivet Wheat (*Triticum turgidum*)
LEADER & HELPER

Country: Middle East
Recommended source: Soul Quintessence System (Leader), Silvercord Essences (Helper)
Combination Essence: Stellaris by Soul Quintessence System (Leader)

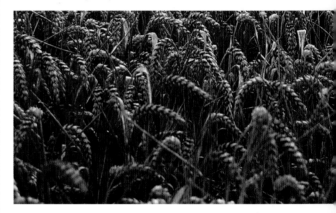

In Essence

A wild, sun-loving straw, Rivet is one of the more primitive forms of wheat, originating around 10,000 years ago. The energy signatures of Avebury Stone Circle and of a crop circle are infused in Soul Quintessence Stellaris essence, as this is where the essence was made. It shows you how to move forward rather than stand at the threshold. Symptoms manifest as excuses as to why you need to take your time – to replace the old you need to shift your consciousness to a broader perspective. This essence removes fear of the unknown and creates broader vision, so that you can do what is necessary with ease. This essence is helpful when dealing with long-standing problems, in unblocking stuck energy – circulation problems, for instance – relieving multidimensional pain and ending procrastination. I find it creates a profound energy increase at the crown chakra and releases old beliefs, limiting confines, entropy and interpersonal conflict, creating inspiration in every aspect of life.

Ti (*Cordyline fruticosa*)
MIMICKER

Alternative names: Cordyline, Good Luck Plant, Hawaiian Ti
Country: Southeast Asia, Papua New Guinea, America (Hawaii), Australia
Recommended source: Gaia Essences

In Essence

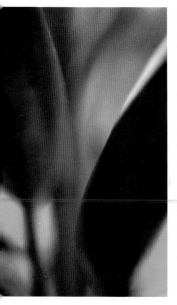

A palm-like evergreen shrub, Ti produces sweetly scented red or yellow flowers and red berries. The leaves are beautiful, thick and lustrous, often splashed with colours from red and pink to copper, which become brighter and more vivid in the sunlight; they are made into traditional Hawaiian 'grass' skirts, so the plant is considered to be a gift of luck. Ti essence strengthens all the energy pathways of the chakras and represents protection, shielding against evil spirits, human or otherwise, and embracing the good. Indeed, the plant is said to help lift curses and has been used by South Pacific islanders for centuries. The essence is good for believers in the power of black magic, helping them shift their focus to a more positive outcome: 'My God, whoever that is, is the best there is – therefore anyone else has no power.'

Soft Rush Grass (*Juncus effusus*)
LEADER

Country: America, Canada, Australia, New Zealand
Recommended source: Silvercord Essences

In Essence

This grass grows in wet cow pastures, along ditches, lake and river margins, and in marshes. Its pale-green stems have no leaves, just a reddish sheath, and can grow over one metre tall. In Japan, the grass is cultivated for tatami, the split-rush flooring. As an essence, it helps with finding new directions and purpose in life. Positive energy helps to increase cross energy to help with the healing process, making it ideal for suffers of chronic arthritis and rheumatism.

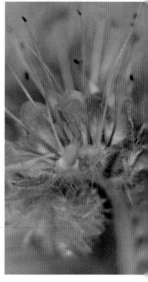

Viper's Bugloss (*Echium vulgare*)
LEADER

Alternative name: Blueweed
Country: Britain, Europe, North America
Recommended source: Korte Essences

In Essence

Viper's Bugloss is a showy plant that grows on walls and in old quarries and gravel pits. Bugloss means ox's tongue, given because of the roughness and shape of the leaves. The plant was once believed to be a remedy against poison, scorpion sting and the bite of a viper – hence the other part of its name. Diuretic and soothing, the leaves alleviate fevers, headaches, nervous complaints and inflammatory pains. The essence helps you develop your warm-hearted side and teaches you that a smile can often open doors; it enables you to recognize that humour and friendliness take you further than a grim sense of duty or discipline.

Olive (Olea europaea)
HELPER AND MIMICKER

Alternative name: Olivier
Country: Portugal, Europe, Mediterranean
Recommended source: Bodylink Essences, Bach Collection by Sun Essences

In Essence

Olive is the oldest known cultivated tree, originating in Africa in 3500 BC. A symbol of wisdom, peace and victory, the goddess Athena is depicted with an Olive branch because she speared the ground, pro-ducing an Olive tree. As an essence, Olive signifies overcoming

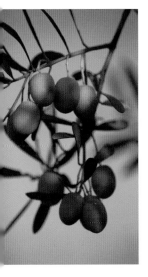

adversity. It is ideal for when life has no joy, there is no light at the end of the tunnel and for exhaustion in all spiritual, mental and physical bodies. Take it when you feel the need to be important to someone else, or for finding a reason to live – it gives us the strength to grow in adversity. Our children learn to rely on us and feed from our knowledge and love; we grow from their reactions, and feed them more. This is an equation of needs being met from both sides, from a reality of love. Olive has been used many times to renew the connection between parents and children, especially in cases of adoption.

Shadow Cactus (Caralluma russelliana)
HELPER

Country: East Africa
Recommended source: Korte Essences

In Essence

An incredible plant, Shadow Cactus has light grey-green stems, with soft ball-sized clusters of dark purple flowers. In essence, Shadow Cactus works on opening the entrance to the subconscious, making it easier to probe into your shadow or dark side. It has a releasing effect on the solar plexus and helps you to see your own shadow and integrate it into your body, to see the dark points in your life and how to work with them positively. You must accept death before you can start with life, and with this essence you can say goodbye to your shadows, accept closure and live in awareness without having to relive any of it. Shadow Cactus also has a balancing effect on the ears.

Scurvy Grass (Cochlearia officinalis)
HELPER

Alternative name: Spoonwort
Country: Britain, Europe
Recommended source: Silvercord Essences

In Essence

Scurvy Grass is a small, low-growing plant, with thick, fleshy, egg-shaped leaves – hence the alternative name of Spoonwort. The leaves have a pungent smell, since they contain sulphur, and a warm, bitter taste. They are stimulating, are diuretic and – not surprisingly, given the plant's name – act against scurvy. So much so, that the fresh herb was historically used on sea-voyages to prevent scurvy and Scurvy Grass ale was a popular tonic drink. In essence, Scurvy Grass helps to cleanse away old memories. It works on the base, sacral and solar plexus chakras, helping to communicate a feeling within that whatever has happened has been and gone, and that it's okay now to move on.

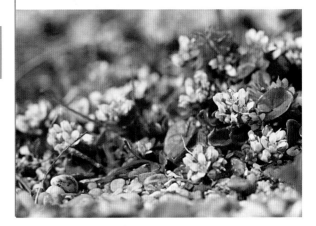

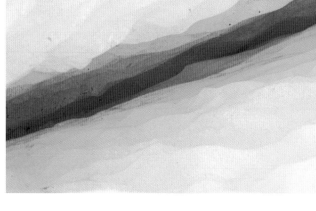

Alpine Bittercress (*Cardamine bellidifolia*)
HELPER

Alternative name: Joklaklukka
Country: North America (Newfoundland to Minnesota, Montana, Florida, Tennessee, Kansas).
Recommended source: Silvercord Essences

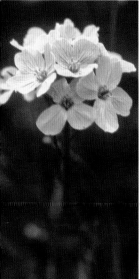

In Essence

Alpine Bittercress is an herbaceous annual with minute white, pink or purple flowers and is much loved by wildlife. The name *Cardamine* is derived from the Greek word *kardamon*, referring to the Persian or Indian herb with pungent, spicy leaves. Reputed as a plant to have medicinal benefits in the treatment of heart or stomach problems, Alpine Bittercress essence helps to release emotional pain from all energy levels. I think that it is an ideal essence for those who need to release and let go of past hurts, and need a bit of love in their lives.

En – (water from the glacial run-off of Jostedalsbreen glacier) LEADER

Country: Norway (Jostedal Glacier National Park)
Recommended source: Bodylink Essences

In Essence

En water is taken from the Jostedalsbreen glacier, which covers almost 190 square miles in the Jostedal National Park. Well-known glacier tongues such as Nigardsbreen, Bergsetbreen, Tuftebreen, Fåbergstølsbreen and Austdalsbreen branch out from this great ice mass, stretching down towards the Jostedalen valley. The glaciers, glacial rivers and moraines, plus the mountain summer pastures, are important preserved landscapes and in many places you can peer into the blue ice of the glacier at very close range. The water is at its purest form in Nature. A pebble thrown into a lake spreads its ripples far and wide; the same thing happens when you are traumatized – even though you can't see them, the ripples are apparent throughout the body long after the original trauma has occurred. En essence works directly on the membrane, removing the ripples from this tidal wave of emotion and trauma and allowing the storm to settle. En can help with guilt issues too.

Cedar (*Cedrus brevifolia*)
HELPER

Alternative names: American Arbor Vitae, Arbor Vitae, Cedrus Lycea, False White Cedar, Hackmatack, Lebensbaum, Thuia du Canada, Tree of Life, Western Arbor Vitae
Country: Himalayas, Mediterranean
Recommended source: Soul Quintessence System

In Essence

This huge, thick, sturdy fir tree produces one of the most beautifully fragrant woods, which has been popular since Egyptian times for perfume and preservation. American Indians believe that the wood

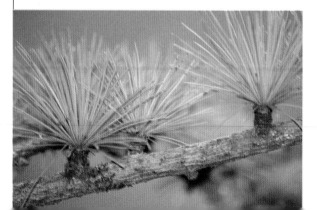

of the Cedar tree holds the powerful protective spirits of ancient ancestors. Its balsamic, camphor-like aroma is still used as the soul of many of today's perfumes and also acts as a moth repellent. Cedar is still placed above the entrances to homes to protect against the entry of evil spirits. The herbal remedy Thuja (a Greek word meaning 'to fumigate', or *thuo* 'to sacrifice') comes from Cedar, since the Ancients burnt its fragrant wood with sacrifices. Cedar essence puts you back in tune with life. It releases boundaries, bondage, prejudice, enslavement and mind programming. An overwhelming opening of the heart is very tangibly experienced when this essence is taken, and physically it helps respiratory and chest problems, when your heart has been dominated and stifled rather than sustained. Healing Hearts – Healing Nations.

Common Wallflower

(Cheiranthus cheiri) HELPER

Alternative names: Baton d'or, Beeflower, Gillyflower, Giroflier, Handflower, Keiri, Wallstock-Gillofer
Country: Britain, Southern Europe
Recommended source: Sovereignty Essences, Gaia Essences
Combined essences: Imbolc Goddess by Sovereignty Essences; Shakti – Sacred Energy by Gaia Essences

In Essence

This homely perennial plant of the cabbage family was introduced into Britain over 300 years ago, and its pretty blooms and delightful fragrance soon made it a cottage garden favourite. It has single yellow-orange flowers, which in olden days were carried in the hands

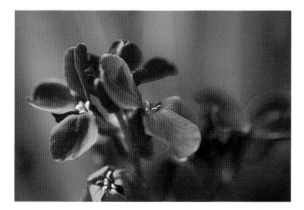

at classic festivals. The plant contains an oil that is part of the digitalis group and it is used in homoeopathy to treat wisdom teeth. The essence is ideal for those who have developed hopelessness and insecurity with an angry twist, always looking for a fight and with a chip on their shoulder. Take inspiration from this loveable flower and seek the positives in life to overfill that empty cup with joy.

Scolecite

HELPER

Country: India
Recommended source: Silvercord Essences

In Essence

Deccan basalt, a common grey to black volcanic rock that flows over 200,000 square miles of the Deccan plateau in west central India, is a prime source of fabulous Scolecite specimens. Large gas bubbles trapped in the solidified lava rock provide ideal sites for the formation of these delicate – and hence extremely valuable – needle-like crystals. Metaphysically, Scolecite is a great team stone. I use it for group-based projects to pull the team together into a more cohesive group and also in offices to engender team spirit; it seems to function as a harmonizing force between different energies, but it also appears to improve communication between people. At a physical level, Scolesite essence helps you to see the truth by removing the cobwebs of illusion, allowing you to focus upon an area that needs to be cleared. Scolesite is like a highly refined tuning fork, helping to realign all the chakras, especially the crown. Its delicate vibrations of ethereal clarity help to loosen and disperse areas of restricted or condensed energy in the mind, body and emotions, creating more space in your consciousness to enable growth and open-mindedness.

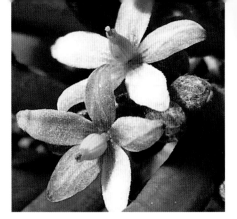

Darnel Grass (*Lolium temulentum*)
HELPER

Alternative names: Ray-grass. Bearded Darnel, Drake, Cheat (*Old English*) Cokil
Country: Britain
Recommended source: Silvercord Essences

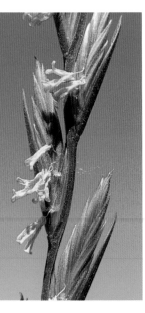

In Essence

A common grass weed in English cornfields, Darnel is virulent and easily distinguished by its long 'glumes' or 'awns'. The seeds or grains were used medicinally by the ancient Greeks and Romans, and it is known for its sedative, relaxing cure for headache, rheumatic meningitis and sciatica. As an essence, Darnel works on the IDA and Pingala meridians. It helps to realign the chakras and helps with life changes, accessing subconscious issues that affect motivation.

Strumpfia (*Strumpfia maritima*)
LEADER, HELPER & MIMICKER

Alternative names: Pride of Big Pine
Countries: Caribbean, North America (southern Florida)
Recommended source: Bodylink Essences

In Essence

Strumpfia is a member of the bedstraw family that can be found growing along rocky coasts and rock gardens by the sea. It has long, needle-like leaves and white to pink showy flowers and is highly resistant to the wind and salinity of the ocean. Its woody stems are often burned as a mosquito repellent and infusions of the leaves are reported to be a nervous stimulant useful in treating poisonous bites, fever, and stupor and weakness caused by fever. As an essence, Strumpfia has

the ability to jump-start and finely tune your protective cross energy – rather like using a defibrillator to restore an otherwise chaotic electrical system. Great in times of emotional and physical fatigue, it restores polarities at certain points, such as ears, jaw, shoulders, elbows, wrists, diaphragm, hips, knees and ankles.

Hawthorn (*Crataegus monogyna*)
LEADER

Alternative names: May, Mayblossom, Quickthorn, Whitethorn, Haw, Hazels, Gazels, Halves, Hagthorn, Ladies' Meat, Bread and Cheese Tree
Country: Europe, North Africa, Western Asia.
Recommended source: Green Man Essences

In Essence

Like its flowers, the Hawthorn fruit, a tiny, bright red apple when ripe, is astringent and an old cure for sore throats. Hawthorn is also used as a cardiac tonic for heart disease and as a diuretic for kidney troubles. As an essence, it helps establish trust and forgiveness, and stimulates the healing power of love. Harbouring a grudge? Hawthorn essence helps cleanse the heart of negativity, so that cross energy is increased at the abdomen, encouraging a smooth flow between the heart and lower body.

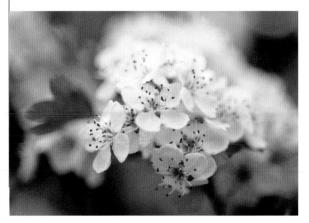

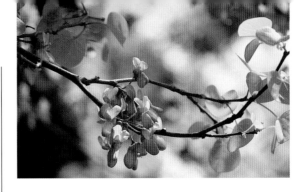

Hyacinth (*Hyacinthus orientalis*)
HELPER

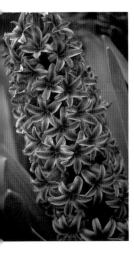

Alternative names: Dutch Hyacinth, Roman Hyacinth
Countries: Mediterranean region (North Africa, Greece), Asia Minor, Syria
Recommended source: Ilminster Essences

In Essence

Stately and sophisticated, the Hyacinth is often grown and given as a gift for its wonderful long-lasting blooms and intoxicatingly sweet scent. According to Homer, the first Hyacinth sprang from the blood of Hyakinthos, the youthful warrior accidentally killed by Apollo. As an essence, Hyacinth works from the base to the crown chakras and helps to 'clear the light.' I find it to be one of the most grounding essences I use on a day-to-day basis (therapists can use it to ground their clients after a massage, too). For those of you who feel as if your energy is everywhere you are not, use Hyacinth to balance the voltage and harmonize your mind, body and soul.

Judas Tree (*Cercis siliquastrum*)
LEADER

Alternative names: Redbud
Countries: Europe, Mediterranean, Asia,
Recommended source: Ilminster Essences

In Essence

The perfect climbing tree, often bent low and hanging to one side, the Judas Tree is certainly ancient; fossils have been found that go back to the Cretaceous period 100 million years ago. Unusually, the flowers not only cover the twigs, but can even sprout from the old bark on the main trunk. In France, it was known as the tree from Judaea (*l'arbre de Judée*); others connect its name to the legend that Judas Iscariot hung himself on such a tree after betraying Christ, hence its deep rosy-red Spring flowers. In essence, the Judas Tree works on all etheric levels to dissolve the shock waves from trauma that are causing guilty feelings. In its role as the 'guilt remover', it aims to restore faith and the spirit of forgiveness; you may find other essences are needed to help support the healing of a trauma. Used in conjunction with En essence, there's nothing better.

Here and Now Cactus
(*Hylocereus undatus*) LEADER

Alternative names: Cactus Pitahaya, Dragon Fruit, Night Blooming Strawberry Pear, Pa-Nani-O-Ka
Countries: Caribbean, southern Mexico, Belize, Guatemala, El Salvador, Costa Rica
Recommended source: Korte Essences

In Essence

An evergreen, vining cactus, the Here and Now Cactus thrives in dry, tropical or subtropical climates. Its extremely fragrant flowers often bloom for just one night, making them in high demand. This is a plant that – thanks to its spines or sharp edges – needs extreme caution when handling; a little like us, perhaps? As a flower essence, it increases cross energy at eye and lower throat level, and enhances your connection with the Earth, a love of nature and your own body, and strengthens your awareness of your energy or aura. Feeling more trusting, you learn to accept your place on Earth, fatalistically.

Indian Fig/Banyan Tree
(Ficus benghalensis) LEADER

Alternative name: Wish-fulfilling Tree
Country: India, Pakistan, Sri Lanka
Recommended source: Soul Quintessence System

In Essence

The Indian Fig or Banyan Tree can grow to huge proportions. It's no surprise that the tree is planted for its shade-giving properties, and historically was used as a 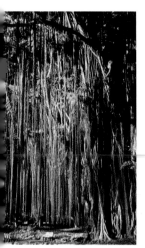 meeting-place for villagers. Fig Tree essence is linked to the memory and the mind, helping to release mental blocks from the subconscious. It inspires integrity – taking this essence helps you to remain true to yourself. The masses are conditioned by mediocrity; we cling to the success of others rather than create it for ourselves, but this breeds unworthiness and envy. There is nothing liberating about playing small so that others feel comfortable. This marvellous essence addresses conformity, superficial behaviour and the blindness created by bureaucracy and politics. It can be challenging to maintain integrity when you are easily swayed by others and are afraid to share your own views – especially if they differ from the consensus. The more you honour your own truth, the more you inspire others to claim their own truth.

Mountain Ash *(Eucalyptus regnans)*
LEADER

Alternative names: Rowan Tree
Country: Europe
Recommended source: Sabian Essences

In Essence

A beautiful tree that grows up high, this is a very spiritual plant. In herbal medicine, the bark of the Mountain Ash helps relieve diarrhoea and the ripe berries make an

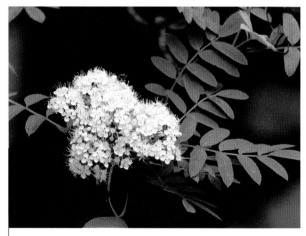

astringent gargle for sore throats and inflamed tonsils. The Mountain Ash affects our high spiritual self. In essence, it stops the energy flow around the spiritual matrix, giving you time off from higher-self talk and allowing you to concentrate, clarify the mind and avoid procrastination. Ideal for those who suffer from a closed mind, clouded vision, an inability to focus or mental imbalances, the Mountain Ash allows an opening to other dimensions, creating a balanced link between body, mind and soul, better focus and mental peace. I find it is useful after surgery, and helpful for post-operative pain.

Tea Rose
(Rosa 'Mr Lincoln') HELPER

Country: North America
Recommended source: Soul Quintessence System
Combined essence: Christ Ray

In Essence

Rosa 'Mr. Lincoln' has an outstandingly strong damask scent that seduces the senses. The beautiful Rose essence from this variety of *Rosa* assists in the birthing of your cosmic self and encourages birthing at all levels. It helps you flow with the biorhythms of the Earth and redress the sins of old with ease and release guilt and shame, promoting forgiveness and atonement.

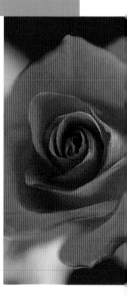

It removes the misconception that you need to suffer to grow, or that you need to take on and carry the burdens of other people. This essence helps you to say goodbye to the sins of old, to guilt, material and spiritual suffering and fear of death, and instead envisage deep healing, conception and birthing at all levels, fertilization at the level of Spirit, resonance and compassionate action. This essence can be used for infertility, for pregnant women prone to miscarriages and for a smooth delivery. It may be useful for regulating biorhythms and for those who wish to birth a new way of being or give birth to a new project.

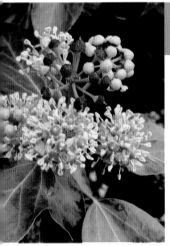

Ivy (*Hedera helix*) LEADER

Alternative name: Common Ivy
Country: Europe, Northern and Central Asia
Recommended source: Gaia Essences, Sovereignty Essences
Combined essences: Demeter – Hope by Gaia Essences; Winter Solstice Goddess by Sovereignty Essences

In Essence

This well-known evergreen climber, with its dark-green, glossy, angular leaves, is nature's most adaptable and steadfast plant. It climbs by means of its roots, which shoot out from every part of the stem, clinging firmly and adapting itself to the roughness of the bark or wall against which it grows. The flowers of the common Ivy are small, yellowish-green clusters. Although they have little or no scent, they are rich in nectar. Ivy was held in high esteem among the ancients – its leaves were used to form the 'poet's crown' as well as the wreath of Bacchus, to whom the plant was dedicated. Greek priests once presented a wreath of Ivy to a newly-married couple, and Ivy has always been regarded as the emblem of fidelity. In essence form, Ivy represents honesty. It balances the heart chakra and its associated nadis. Take the essence to ease hidden fears and anxieties; it helps to release true feelings and identify your emotional needs.

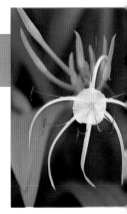

Spider Lily (*Hymenocallis littoralis*) LEADER & HELPER

Alternative name: Beach Spider lily
Country: East Asia (China, Japan)
Recommended source: Bodylink Essences (Leader), Gaia Essences (Helper)

In Essence

This tropical plant, with its lovely white, heavily scented flowers, has been known since ancient times to possess anti-tumour activity, mainly due to the component lycorine, which has antineoplastic and antiviral properties – research is under way to study its benefit in the treatment of HIV. Energetically, Spider Lily essence helps eliminate depression in the spiritual matrix – it says 'pull yourself together,' thereby releasing chains or clearing up loose ends. A great essence, which really helps you to hold yourself together in a stressful situation.

Gardenia (*Gardenia jasminoides*) LEADER, HELPER & MIMICKER

Alternative names: Cape Jasmine, Common Gardenia
Country: China
Recommended source: Gaia Essences
Combined essence: Mary – Purification by Gaia Essences

In Essence

The fragrant Gardenia flower is hugely popular in perfumery. The root is used to help headaches, dyspepsia, nervous disorders and fever, and the fruits have been used for jaundice and kidney and lung disorders. Gardenia essence represents death and dying. It clears the contacts between body and spirit for easy release – not always death itself, but a significant life change. It's for moving on through a cycle, and is invaluable for people who can't let go of unrewarding jobs or relationships. This essence helps you to surrender to the inevitable and stop resisting a peaceful transition.

Chapter 4

How to Use Flower Essences

There's a way for everyone to feel comfortable taking an essence, from ingesting drops in brandy, vodka or spring water, to taking a flower-essence bath or spraying your aura. It's your choice.

Under the Tongue

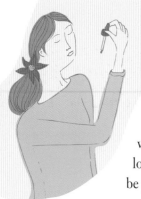

Below:
Essences can be dropped under the tongue for fast absorption.

The most common way to take essences is sublingually, or droplets under the tongue, which are quickly absorbed into the bloodstream and transported around the body, bringing a rapid beneficial effect. Medication for the symptoms of angina is taken this way, for fast, effective relief of pain. Taking your essence under the tongue is also a speedy and efficient way of getting it into the cells of your body. It is not always possible to get drops under the tongue when giving an essence to children and in this case any way is better than no way, as long as the essence goes inside the mouth. Most essences are preserved in alcohol – either vodka or brandy; vodka is preferable because it doesn't taint the essence. If you do not want an alcoholic preservative, essences can be preserved in organic cider vinegar or vegetable glycerine. Most children's essences are stored in glycerine (children love it) and animals also like their essences in glycerine, although the drops can be placed in their food to ensure the full dose is taken.

Spring-Water 'Shot'

You can add the essence drops to a small amount of spring water and drink the mixture. Many clients opt for this method as they can count the number of drops more easily than when dropping the essence directly into the mouth. You may also find essences prepared as a mouth spray – they are usually designed for easy application when you are on the move and not able to count drops.

Topical Application

Many therapists recommend applying the essence directly onto a pulse point, usually on the wrist. Of course this is not recommended if the preparation has been made up in glycerine, as it will make your skin sticky. You can even get essences supplied in a convenient rollerball applicator. You can also add an essence to a cream (such as vitamin E cream), or in cooling aloe vera gel – ideal for those with psoriasis. Put the drops in the cream before you rub it into your skin: the essence is readily absorbed by the skin and the capillaries feeding blood to the area, thereby ensuring assimilation into your aura (your energy field). Essences are great wound healers too, both physical and emotional, especially when an injury is not healing properly or is taking too long to heal, or to prevent a scar from becoming keloid. Apply only after the wound has closed, and on scars. Orange essence cream is particularly good, with added Water Moss and Star of Bethlehem. When the skin has been broken – for example, by a surgical incision – you have in effect broken your body's outer protection barrier and the body will be working overtime to reinforce its physical shield and fight off any possible intrusion from bacteria. The body is so clever, but unfortunately your emotions play a huge part in just how quickly or slowly you recover from the trauma of surgery, so you need to help your emotional self readjust to this trauma as well.

Below:
Star of Bethlehem is a wonderful wound-healer.

Case Study

John accidentally amputated his finger whilst performing some DIY and also sustained numerous cuts to his other three fingers. His finger was rejoined, but it required three operations – quite a traumatic event to anyone. I met him in casualty at his local hospital to give him Reiki and Stress Buster essence , which helped to deal with the initial shock, but as his recovery progressed it became clear the keloidosis was taking over the entire scarring. He applied Orange essence in a cream to the scars once the skin was healed and over a period of three months, the scarring reduced to fine lines with no residual keloid scarring.

Misting

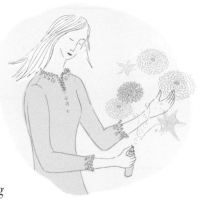

Right:
*You can apply essences
like perfume – dilute
in water and mist
your pulse points.*

Many essences are designed to be sprayed and they
usually come in a mister bottle ready for use.
These often include a number of essential oils to
give a pleasant aroma and work with the essences,
to help the process of change. It is important to
note that essential oils are not flower essences or
vibrational essences (see page 27), and are not made
in the same way. If you are using sprays containing
essential oils when you are pregnant please take the same precautions that you
would when using any essential oil(s) because of the potentially toxic nature of
some of them, and always check the label to confirm any sensitivity.

Protecting your Aura

A sprayed essence hits the aura (the energy field) and is instantly absorbed from
the outside in, so it is a very effective way of using essences. This method is perfect
when you need to protect your personal space, for instance in dental surgeries,
hospitals, and while travelling on airplanes, buses or trains. A protection spray is
essential for your personal energy integrity – think of your aura fighting for the
same space as hundreds of other auras, which is why we can pick up the emotions
of others as easily as picking up airborne bugs. If you travel a great deal and find
that you are susceptible to picking up colds and snuffles on planes, think about
what your energy field is picking up at the same time. You can also pick up feelings
of panic and anxiety before and while flying, whereas spraying an essence can instil
a sense of calm and space.

Case Study

Tom was recently in hospital for a heart bypass operation. The whole energy of a
hospital is one of infirmity; people are sick and negative, trying to deal with the
emotions of fear and anxiety for all sorts of reasons, and there's very little positive
energy. It's one of the reasons why people dread going to hospital and people

instinctively take flowers to give to their friends and relatives. Unfortunately, Intensive Care is one place where flowers are not allowed, although it is probably the place you need flower essences the most. Having worked in an Intensive Care Unit, I know first-hand how much these patients need support, care and compassion. I sprayed Tom's ICU room with En for trauma, Heliconium for fear, Frangipani for healing and White Mangrove for nurture. When Tom moved out of the Intensive Care Unit, I changed the flower essence spray to Olive, Lemon, Casuarina Flowers and Love in a Mist. This essence is cleansing for the emotional outpouring after such surgery, helping the bones to heal, giving a feeling of being loved and cared for, and encouraging an optimistic attitude to being fit and feeling good. His medical team were surprised at how quickly Tom recovered, and he was discharged early.

Left:
Love in a Mist can help release emotions and encourage healing.

Misting your Environment

An essence used as a room spray enhances the negative ions around you and your environment, at home or work. You may want to achieve specific goals within your space – for instance, increased love, prosperity or security. Just think about hotel rooms: how many have you stayed in and because they are so impersonal you make a mess to put your stamp on them? I recommend a cleansing spray, such as Pine or Horsetail She-Oak essence, when travelling – many long-haul flight staff wouldn't go without one. Don't go anywhere? Then look closer to home. On average a house has three to four occupants, so what are the chances that everyone is having a great day? How do you stop that black cloud coming out of your teenager's room and engulfing the whole house? Simple – use the cleansing spray. You can get a personal home blend of essences specially for your home from Intuits™ (see page 141). Decant the dose into a spray of spring water to mist in and around your home every day to achieve the desired effect. This is especially recommended for areas affected by electromagnetic fields from computers, televisions and radios.

Below:
Horsetail She-Oak as an essence is a great cleanser – mist hotel rooms to neutralize old energy.

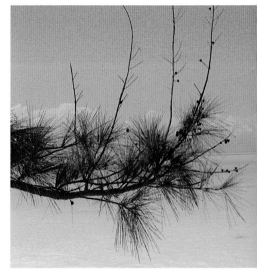

Case Study

A female client of mine, who was receiving treatment for another matter, happened to mention that she was also having a very challenging time at work. She had the overwhelming task of closing the business down and making the entire staff redundant. The management team were expecting the worst, and the lawyers and HR team had booked an entire day out to deal with it. I recommended peace-making Lamium essence, for change, and for its conciliatory effect. She sprayed the meeting room beforehand, then added a few drops to the drinking water for the participants of the meeting. She rang me later to say that the meeting was over amicably within an hour.

Baths and Footbaths

Below:
You can add a few drops of your chosen essence(s) to bath water.

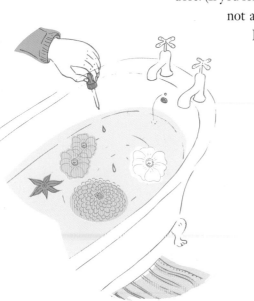

Any essence can be placed in the bath or in a footbath. After all, flower essences naturally work through the resonance of water, and it's a gentle way to use essences for physical traumas such as childbirth, fractures, mental and physical abuse and accidents – especially for children. If using an essence in the bath, don't take your normal oral dose that evening or morning, otherwise you would be doubling the dose. (If you forget, don't worry – you may cry a few tears and maybe that's not a bad thing, as crying is a release and cleanses the system. Even boys do it!) Make a ceremony of adding essences to the bath water – a few lit candles strategically placed around the bathroom and soft music enhance your mood of receptivity and relaxation, and enable the essence to do its job with relative ease. Let yourself relax into the healing vibrations of the essences as they seep directly into your aura and physical body. As blockages are cleared, visualize your unwanted emotions swirling down the drain. An instant lift!

Frequently Asked Questions

Can I use more than one essence at a time?

Several flower essences can be taken together (ideally no more than four essences at any one time, unless you are working with a skilled practitioner) mixed together in a dosage bottle, then used daily via one of the methods mentioned on pages 88–92. When making your own combined essence, it is important to consider which essences work in harmony together and support each other's actions. For instance: Bay Cedar for protection and stability; Aaron's Rod, for courage and conviction; Seaside Centaury for clarity. Obviously using an essence to help you express your emotions would not be most effective if it is combined with an essence for drying up the tears.

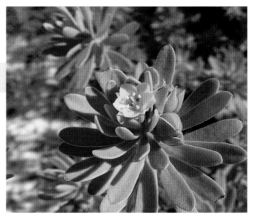

Above:
Bay Cedar flower essence gives protection and stability.

How do I get the maximum benefit from using flower essences?

Flower essences work best when one is open and receptive. You may find that a quiet space, free from distraction, and perhaps creating time for a little meditation, will boost the effects. Often people taking flower essences on a regular basis find that they become more aware of their diet and the stresses in their life and develop the need for a little 'me-time'. However, you don't have to 'believe' in the benefits for an essence to work, other than having a willingness to try them. Children and animals have no preconceived ideas about essences one way or the other and they always show the benefits. People from a wide range of cultures, backgrounds and lifestyles have benefited from their use, with excellent results. I always suggest that my clients keep a journal – buy a cheap exercise book and date and time your entries. You don't have to make it a diary – just a line or two is great, or even a one-word entry as long as you know what it means. Sometimes the effects of essences are lost in the everyday ravages of life and you may not notice a difference until the end of a two- or four-week period. Then a song you hear on the radio may prompt a response that reminds you of an event or person from long ago.

This may be integral to your healing process and may be the catalyst needed to open the floodgates. Write it all down – it's also helpful to get it out of your head, where it has no escape but simply goes round and round. Putting it on paper allows you to read and reread your entries and see the patterns that are emerging.

Is every flower remedy effective for me?

Flower essences work by a principle of resonance. They will be most effective and noticeable when they actually match the core mental or emotional challenges you face and can specifically pinpoint for yourself at any given time – such as fear of flying, procrastination, uncertainty and anxiety. If you are addressing only surface symptoms, or fleeting feelings, you may not notice much impact from the flower essences – although the effect will most definitely be there. Think of your house with its miles and miles of electrical wiring: if you have a problem with the main light in your kitchen you call the electrician and he either repairs or replaces it. We can't do that with the body, so we have to try and pinpoint where the fault is and then match it with the essence that works there. This sends out a vibration that resonates with exactly the right match and, 'hey presto!' the light's back on. The most important thing to remember is that if you choose the wrong essence it will simply do nothing.

Above:
Betony flower essence relaxes your attitude so you become more receptive.

How will flower essences make me feel?

In the long run, working with flower essences will help you to feel more energetic, vibrant, positive, focused and 'in touch' with your goals, morals and personal creativity. Essences do not, however, create euphoria, nor do they banish pain and conflict. They work by stimulating awareness of inner conflicts and challenges, thereby strengthening our ability to work through any obstacles to our total fulfilment in life, health and wisdom. Taking flower essences may, at times, stimulate some emotional discomfort and stark awareness of deep-seated pain or discord. It is important to remember that this is a normal part of any journey towards wellness, and will ultimately lead to a much more complete state of health than the suppression of pain, or the artificial stimulation of feelings through drugs, painkillers, antidepressants, or other biochemical intervention. Essences work with the body's natural flow rather than against it, so it may take a little longer than you would like – but the results will be longer-lasting.

Can I use flower essences if I am on medication?

Yes, most definitely, although you should be aware that when on antidepressants or anti-anxiety medication it can be very difficult to feel the changes taking place. This does not mean that they are not happening, so persevere.

Can I use flower essences if I am an alcoholic/recovering alcoholic?

Of course, but I think it's imperative that alcohol is avoided as a preservative. Essences can also help to relieve the addictive tendencies exhibited by those suffering from dependent urges.

Do flower essences have physical effects?

Flower essences do not work biochemically, as an aspirin does for a headache, but they do affect our experience of our bodies. For example, essences such as Alder, Lamium and Lime (citrus), which help release emotional stress, may result in less physical tension. Someone who overworks may take Couch Grass and only then discover just how tired they really are. Flower essences help those of us with a very real physical illness by addressing the emotional responses to the illness, and by working with the underlying conflicts and tensions that may have contributed to its onset in the first place. However, flower essences are not cures, and if you are suffering from a serious medical complaint they should be used in conjunction with consultation from a qualified health practitioner. Many health practitioners now include flower essences in their health programmes, or work with other complementary practitioners who do.

How should I look after my flower essences?

Flower essences are usually stored and dispensed in a dark glass bottle to prevent oxidation by sunlight and to keep the essence integral. You will need to store the bottle where you can see it, just as a reminder – but don't leave it by a clock-radio or computer where it can be affected by emissions. You must remember that the essence is a living product and can be adversely affected by its environment. One client couldn't understand why her essence wasn't doing anything for her when her friend was having amazing results. 'What am I doing wrong, am I not taking the right essence?' she asked. The first question elicited the reason: she kept the bottle on a radiator and it's certainly not a good idea to cook the flowers. If you carry your essence in your handbag, do not keep it by a mobile phone and if you leave it in a car, remember how hot a car gets in sun. Storing your essence by your bed is a good reminder to take it first thing in the morning and last thing at night, but note that the phone and clock shouldn't be within reaching distance of it.

One-dosage bottle of 15ml should last you two weeks with regular use, and keep for about three months, providing it is preserved in alcohol – but it will last for much less time if preserved in glycerine. If you do have the glycerine alternative, bear in mind that bugs love to grow in sweet liquids so if you touch the dropper with your mouth, always rinse and sterilize it in boiling water before replacing it in the bottle. This is a really important point to remember when dosing your animals with flower essences, as they have the worst dental hygiene and their mouths are full of gremlins.

When should I take essences?

I like to suggest that essences are taken 15 minutes after or before food, cleaning the teeth, smoking or drinking fluids other than water. This gives a clear pathway for them to work, rather than having to get through the energy of other substances before finding a clear road ahead. It's also nice to make a ceremony out of it – it helps to give the essence a sacred space to work from and make the process special, rather than just popping pills and giving over your energy to another substance. In this way you are part of the process.

Right:
Blue Iris essence helps you find the pathway to your spiritual needs.

Essence Safety

To keep your essence in good condition, always store it away from heat and light and not within reaching distance of appliances that may affect its healing vibrations, such as telephones, televisions or computers. Remember to take your dose, morning and night. It doesn't matter if you take too much, but if you don't take enough the healing process will not be as fast as you might like.

Essences are quite safe for children – even babies – and for animals. Make sure essences for them are made up in glycerine rather than alcohol. If you accidently touch the dropper to a child's or animal's mouth, clean and sterilize it carefully before returning to the bottle so bacteria do not get the chance to multiply.

Do not take more than four essences at once, unless they have been prescribed by an experienced practitioner. Remember that some essential oils are toxic, so if your essence has been added to an essential oil for massage or in a spray, be very careful to follow all instructions as to how and when you can use it.

Above:
St John's Wort is a fabulous essence for quiet, shy types who need to be more assertive.

Top Tips for Taking Essences

- Make a ceremony of taking your essence – it will make you more receptive to the beneficial effect
- Taking your essence under the tongue is fast and efficient
- Adding drops to spring water means they are easy to count
- Mouth sprays or roller applicators are useful when you are on the move
- Add your essence to a footbath or bath, as a gentle and soothing way to use it for traumas
- Essences added to cooling aloe vera gel are great for those with psoriasis
- Use essences to help scars heal and prevent them turning keloid
- Protect your aura in crowded or hostile environments by spraying essence
- If you don't want an alcoholic preservative, essences can be preserved in organic cider vinegar or vegetable glycerine
- Don't apply flower essences preserved in glycerine to the skin – it will make you sticky

Giving Children Essences

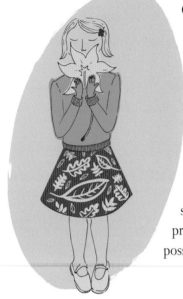

Children and animals typically progress faster than adults when using vibrational essences. This is because they have fewer layers of character and defences built up over time, in response to the wounds that we all experience throughout our lives. However, if children have been abused or abandoned – if their wounds are deep so you are not just using essences to address typical developmental issues – this is not the case, and additional forms of therapy are strongly advised.

Flower and vibrational essences may be used for a great many situations, problems and goals with children – pretty much anything you can think of! Nightmares, bedwetting, shyness, social, learning and school issues, neediness, daydreaming, hypersensitivity, fears, bonding problems, abuse, abandonment and trauma are just some of the possibilities. These issues are included in the charts on pages 125–126.

Essences for Children

Children usually love taking vibrational essences. The bottles containing the essences (for children, usually in glycerine) may be decorated with stars or stickers to personalize them, and you can create lovely affirmations to be used with a child when taking the drops, so it becomes a special time.

If a baby is still nursing, it will receive any essences the mother is taking through the mother's milk. Since the mother may influence the child's behaviour and responses it will almost certainly be beneficial to give the essences to both at the same time. By agreeing to take the essence you are already opening up to its healing vibrations – they are not confined to the little bottle they are in; the energy of the essences permeates the surrounding area as well, just as it does with your own body. I see it all the time in my shop, Essence World. We have over one thousand essences sitting in a very small area and everyone feels the energy of the vibrations as soon as they walk in.

Right:
Cyclamen helps release deep-seated trauma.

How to Give Children Essences

The best way to administer essences to a child is in the mouth, but if this is not possible there are other ways to give the drops:

- Massage on in creams with added essential oils
- Add to the child's food or drink
- Give essences to a baby by rubbing them on its wrists
- Dab the essence behind the ears
- Dab the essence on the forehead
- Add to the child's bath water
- Place a bottle of essence under a baby's crib (safely out of reach) – this will have an effect simply through the vibrations

Essences and ADD or ADHD

There has been a great deal of work on using flower essence therapy with children who have been diagnosed as having Attention Deficit Disorder (ADD) and Attention Deficit Hyperactivity Disorder (ADHD). It has been found that, in the majority of cases, children suffering from these disorders experienced some trauma stemming from early childhood.

My first son, Stuart, cried like mad all the time from birth, and when he had his first triple antigen he collapsed. The remainder of his inoculations were given in quarter doses but from then on he was a complete nightmare in his behaviour. When he was diagnosed with ADHD, the doctor/Homoeopath actually put it down to the effect of the inoculations! When the trauma is treated with flower essences, combined with other forms of therapy, the symptoms associated with ADD and ADHD often decrease or disappear. However, it is most helpful if parents are willing to consider dietary issues that may also be a contributing factor.

Above:
White yarrow essence helps maintain personal boundaries.

Giving Animals Essences

Essences may be helpful for animals in many ways, among them in rescue work, in preparation for surgery and as a healing aid and support during physical illness. They are also useful for fears, grief, separation anxiety, depression, tension, stress, emotional upset, jealousy, mother-infant bonding, socialization issues, aggression, abuse, hyperactivity, aloofness and apathy, and to aid in training or adjusting to new situations. One practitioner I know has reported that when epileptic animals are treated with an emergency or rescue formula, the severity of the attack decreases, the length of the attack is shortened, and attacks happen less frequently. Sometimes pets take on the emotions of their caretakers or are affected by their caretakers' emotions. In cases such as this, relief for the animal may only be possible when the caretaker also takes essences and tries to work with his or her own emotional issues. Some cases are only resolved when both the caretaker and pet are involved with flower essence therapy. Some essence makers recommend that the caretaker and animal both take the same essence or blend in order to improve bonding and to create a mutual resonance between them, which facilitates healing.

How to Give Animals Essences

The best way to administer essences to an animal is by mouth, under the tongue, rubbed into the gums or in their food. If placing the essences directly into the mouth is not possible, you may, as an alternative, place the drops:

- On a treat (dog biscuits, slices of apple, carrots, etc.)
- In the pet's food or water
- On the pads of the paws

- Behind the ears
- On the forehead
- In the pet's bath water
- On a spot the animal will lick

Other Alternatives

Other alternatives for administering essences to animals include gently rubbing the chosen essences onto the palms of your hands, and then applying them through petting the animal – this is very enjoyable for small animals such as hamsters, guinea pigs and mice, as well as for cats and dogs.

Birds are very sensitive to touch so you may prefer to give them essences, with no added preservative, dropped onto the tip of the beak, or you may want to add them to a bowl of water near the bird's cage, so that they will evaporate into the surrounding air. I prefer simply to mist the bird's cage, or mist the air about three feet above the bird.

Some animals with tough skin, such as snakes, like the essences rubbed onto their bodies; and you may also add essences to their water. My family put essences in Mitch the snake's water, which he likes to bathe in, or onto the mice he eats.

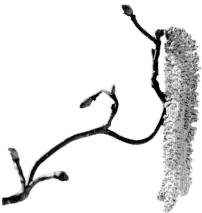

Above:
Hazel essence is helpful for clearing energy debris from the soles of the feet. It is also a great essence for animals.

Choosing Essences for Animals

Obviously, animals cannot tell you what the problem is, so it can be difficult to decide which essence to try. This is where Intuits™ for animals are perfect; they are easily chosen by the owner, with amazing success. For further help in defining the problem, see the chart of symptoms on pages 130–131 and 133–135.

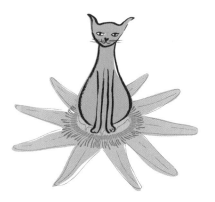

Chapter 5

Symptoms, Causes and Flower Remedies

How to Use the Flower Essence Symptom Finder

Finding a definitive essence for a physical problem can often be quite difficult, as we are so different in our makeup and in the variety of physical and emotional incidents that happen to us through our lives, forming our identity as an individual and making us unique. For instance, in general, breast cancer is a physical result of an emotional response to anger at not being nurtured, but this anger can be at yourself or at others. Some people appear to be an angel to everyone around them, but their emotions are hidden deep inside, locked away for no-one else to see – and often they may not even recognize the anger in themselves. Those around them might say: 'It's not fair, she's such a lovely person, never has a bad word to say about anyone.' – when in fact, she's a very good actress and covers up her true feelings very well. Believe me, I know this first-hand – I left a relationship after a very long time because I couldn't keep up the pretence anymore. I was aching all over and had found a lump in my breast (which turned out to be nothing, thank goodness) and I was extremely unhappy just recognizing the truth. Everyone I knew couldn't believe the situation: 'But you are so happy. You of all people? I thought this was a fairytale relationship.' I've also heard many times how it's really unjust that all the bad people never get sick and the lovely people are often ill, but there is always a reason for chronic disease such as cancer and arthritis. If it isn't apparent on the surface, I can guarantee that there's definitely something buried deep down inside.

Below:
Snowdrop essence can help with respiratory problems.

Emotional Issues

One's reasons for anything are very much one's own, but we can generalize and say, for instance, that an overall emotional aspect is anger, resentment or frustration. It is often said that we also choose our parents. Many of my clients have snorted in derision at this statement, and you may well be doing the same right now! Please, don't discount this – by closing the door on help to relieve your symptoms you are ultimately going it alone. There is so much help all around us that it is foolhardy to think we know the truth, just because of an acquired and rigid mental process, so humour me. This rigid thinking, may, after all, be the very cause of your symptoms.

Below:
Birch essence can help with itchy skin, and its underlying cause – sadness and itching for change.

Let's say, for instance, that I need to learn in my life to stand up for myself, and say, 'No, don't hurt me. I deserve better. I'm not going to let you, by words or actions, hurt and abuse me.' Would you be better served having parents who are perfect, or parents who help you to achieve this life path by giving you an opportunity to say this? If I want to believe that someone is out to get me, I become angry, controlled, and victimized and take the path of blockage and pain. However, if I choose the viewpoint that this person is only showing me my faults, I am empowered to change the situation and do something about it. Try it. If it works, does it really matter who is right or wrong, when you are the winner because you have no pain, emotionally or physically?

The road to health is a long one but, hey, we have all our lives to achieve it. It can be a happy process or a sad one – it's your choice. It's the same when we learn to read, write or integrate into a new job – we listen to our mentors because they have been down this path before and know the easiest route to help us do it better.

Changes and Challenges

Ailments are simply symptoms of our inability to accept the changes and challenges we are presented with, due to our unique history or the personality that we have adapted over the years. All we have to do is be honest and true to ourselves, realize our weaknesses and then have the courage to turn a negative into a positive. I have personally found that if I know what the problem is, then it is much easier to change it. The beauty is that, with the help of flower essences, this becomes a much easier process than if you are attempting it all on your own. Think of it as a journey, helped along by a trusted friend, holding your hand and leading the way.

Physical Symptoms

Energy medicine is complementary help to your wellbeing. Our history causes our symptoms and if you have very physical symptoms you must surely do all you can to alleviate the problem. When the disease process has gone too far and has affected the physical tissue and it needs excising, cut it out if that is what is required, but please do all you can to help ensure that it doesn't reappear or get any worse by looking at the reason for it being there in the first place. When you realize you have the power to do something about your situation you are empowered, not disempowered. Energetically this keeps you positive and moving in the right direction, rather than stagnating and allowing those blockages to manifest or worsen.

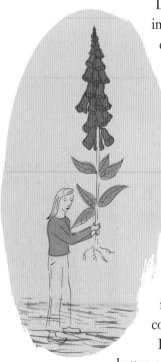

Below:
Foxglove essence can help treat anxiety.

Louise Hay, the well-known author of many books on the subject including *You Can Heal your Life*, is a master of the metaphysical cause of disease. I personally have used her references for many years and the majority of complementary therapists use this work as their bible. Why? Because it works. For instance, I recently had my briefcase, which contained years and years of work on essences, stolen. It was at the end of a brilliant day and life was great, so the moment I realized the magnitude of the situation, I said aloud, 'I will not allow you to spoil my happiness, it must need rewriting.' Driving home, I noticed a pain in my jaw but I remained calm and tried to relax the muscles. As the evening went on, the pain got worse and worse to the point where my jaw was now locked in place. Finally I said aloud, 'Okay, Louise. What do you have to say about this?' The answer – anger and the desire for revenge, with jaw tightly shut, clamped by my own muscles. I muttered, 'Louise, you are so right.' While on the surface I was dealing with the intrusion of my space and the stealing of my property, underneath my cool exterior I was festering with anger and resentment.

I then took a concoction of essences, slept it off, and woke feeling much better, although still a little tender from the ordeal. You see, the only one being hurt in this scenario was me and I wasn't going to let the incident get the better of me. My feelings were hurting me and the only way to let the pain go was to see that. Honour and recognize how you feel: you can't put a bandage on it – it won't go away.

Intuitively Prescribing

The list of ailments and appropriate flower essences here is a great guide. The first column shows your symptom, the second the reason or the emotion you are feeling – in other words, where you are now, or where you want to be – the third shows the recommended Flower Leader and the last a selection of possible Helpers. While I can give an appropriate essence for the symptom listed, I cannot wholly identify the support or flower helper you would need to deal with the issue 100 percent. This is because I cannot make any assumptions about each individual's cause for their response to the problems presented – we are all unique and we deal with our problems as our history dictates. So this is where you come in: one of the reasons my Intuits™ system was developed (see page 141) was to encourage each individual to choose intuitively what they needed to support a change in themselves. You know your body better than anyone else; you just need a way to block out the stuff that gets in the way of your intuition. Without the Intuits™ system, you can use the formula here to choose your own unique mix of essences. You can browse the listings and choose the appropriate Leader (a maximum of two), then a Helper. To personalize this, close your eyes, focus on the centre of your chest and ask, 'What do I need to help this process?' Let your intuition guide you. Open the book, choose the left or right page and point at the paper still with closed eyes. What does it say? Is it relevant to your life? Good luck and happy hunting!

Left:
Gardenia essence can help with the process of bereavement.

Below:
Wild Cherry essence helps calm emotional pain.

Essences for Adults

Symptom	Reason/Emotion (How you are now – where you want to be)	Flower Leader	Flower Helper
Abdominal pains	Fear (*see Pain*)	Heliconium	Sun Orchid
Aches and pains	Inertia, wishing, longing and hoping for a change but doing nothing about it	Blackberry	Sun Orchid Golden Rutilated Quartz
Addictions (alcoholism)	Indicates trauma to the base chakra, which creates an imbalance to fight-and-flight response and a dependence on chaos and addictions	Horsetail She-Oak Flamboyant Tree Star of Bethlehem	Citrine Golden Rutilated Quartz
Allergies (sensitivities)	Oversensitivity, irritability	Bay Cedar Alder	Geranium
Alzheimer's, dementia, senility	I want to live in my own world. Refusing to see the real picture	Centaurea	Isis Lady's Smock Pine
Anorexia/bulimia	Loathing of self, because of a belief in others' views of yourself. A need to control	Birch	Mary Geranium Golden Rutilated Quartz
Anxiety	Lack of trust in self and others. Not listening to inner self	Lamium Foxglove	Peace Nostrum
Apathy	Needing a reason to live, fear of being a part of life	Blackberry Lammas	Darnel Grass Olive Athena Hyacinth Blue
Appetite – excessive	Fear (*see Pain*) Internal protection	Christ Ray	Water Lily
– loss of	No vision for the future	Mountain Ash	Stargazer Lily
Arthritis/joints	Resentment and bitterness	Lemon Bakul Tree Soft Rush Grass Christ Ray	Demeter Italian Arum Maize

Symptom	Reason/Emotion (How you are now – where you want to be)	Flower Leader	Flower Helper
Asthma	Stifled, mothering, smothering	Lamium Passion Flower Cedar Sunset	Motherwort Cedar Golden Rutilated Quartz
Back – upper – middle – lower	Support Lack of emotional support Lack of confidence to support self Lack of financial support	Flame Tree Lime (Linden) Green Alkanet	Water Lily Rowan
Bad breath (halitosis)	Anger, feelings of revenge, 'stinking thinking'	Banyan Tree	Hathor Heather Rowan
Bell's Palsy	Anger at not being able to express oneself	Peace Nostrum	Star of Bethlehem Venus Orchid
Birth process – fertility – safe and happy labour – post-partum	Trusting in the outcome Expectations (for both partners) Letting go Changing cycles, loss of control	Black Wattle Christ Ray Blackberry Blackberry	Motherwort Athena/Rowan Demeter Rose Rowan
Blood pressure problems – high – low	Both long-term issues Relating to emotional pain and retreat Relating to futility of life, usually from childhood	Foxglove Hawthorn Heart to Heart	Hellebore Demeter
Blood problems – anaemia, clotting	Life force issues. Emotional stagnation, can't find the way forward, giving up	Soft Rush Grass Victoria Regia Casuarina Flowers	Winter Solstice
Body odour	Over-aggressive, false over-confidence. Secondary second chakra problems from over-use supporting the base chakra	Silver Princess	Purple Iris
Boils	Anger coming to boiling point	Passion Flower	Heather Common Wallflower
Bowels – constipation – diarrhoea – IBS	Processing of information, either flushing out or holding onto	Blackberry Flamboyant Tree	Timothy Grass Clay Rowan

Symptom	Reason/Emotion (How you are now – where you want to be)	Flower Leader	Flower Helper
Breast cancer	Deep hidden resentment at not being nurtured	Ivy Passion Flower	Mary Demeter Winter Solstice
Breast problems (cysts, mastitis, breast cancer, lumps)	A need for nurture and care, most probably from oneself	Snowdrop Iolite	Oak Cedar Demeter Mary Marsh Helleborine Heart to Heart Heather Thistle
Breathing problems (panic attacks, hyperventilation)	Do I deserve to exist? Frustration, no help available	Lamium Lime (Citrus) Cedar Sunset	Cedar Heart to Heart
Bruises	Needing to punish the self	Christ Ray En Orange Judas Tree	Pine Heart to Heart
Burns	Anger	Horsetail She-Oak Passion Flower	Imbolc Lilac Common Wallflower
Bursitis (frozen shoulder, tennis elbow, clenched fists at night)	Anger, wanting to hit out. Secondary to fear, base chakra secret wanting to speak out	Peace Nostrum Blue Gum Passion Flower	Venus Orchid Maize Common Wallflower Beltane
Circulation	Withdrawing from life	Bakul Tree Cedar Sunset	Demeter Rowan Heather Water Moss
Cold sores	Blistered words	Cedar Sunset Peace Nostrum	Heather Clay Blue Spirea Lilac
Colds	Too much going on, internal crying	Peace Nostrum Blackberry	Marsh Helleborine Quaking Grass Lilac
Colic	Impatient, constant annoyance	Buddleia Butterfly	Purple Toadflax

Symptom	Reason/Emotion (How you are now – where you want to be)	Flower Leader	Flower Helper
Cramps	Fear and tension	Heliconium Buddleia Butterfly Red River Gum Silver Banksia	Imbolc Oak Star of Bethlehem
Crying (despondency)	Release of pent-up sadness. Remember, crying is good, but don't let it take over your life: pity parties can only be attended by one – you. They are boring to other people	White Mangrove	Marsh Helleborine Peace Nostrum Olive Frangipani
Cuts and grazes	Self-punishment	Orange	Water Moss Star of Bethlehem
Cystitis	Being 'peed off'	Flame Tree Horsetail She-Oak	Maize Scurvy Grass Rowan Orange Azalea Purple Toadflax Sand Rush Grass
Death and dying	Cycle is finished, contract is over, helping to accept the process and to smooth the path	Heart to Heart Gardenia Victoria Regia Christ Ray Heliconium Cedar Sunset	Forget-Me-Not Heather Italian Arum Rowan
Depression	Despondent, unable to change and anger at the self	Spider Lily St John's Wort Black Wattle	Velvet Bentgrass
Diabetes	Bitter, no sweetness in one's life, not taking responsibility for one's actions	Silver Banksia Centaurea	Star of Bethlehem Velvet Bentgrass European Spindle Tree Lammas Athena Rowan
Endometriosis	Low self-esteem and self-love	Silver Princess Red River Gum St John's Wort	Isis Grounding Opuntia Cactus
Epilepsy	Life is a battle – an inability to cope	Blackberry Centaurea	Rowan Hyacinth Blue

SYMPTOM	REASON/EMOTION (How you are now – where you want to be)	FLOWER LEADER	FLOWER HELPER
Eye problems (conjunctivitis, dry eye, cataracts, eye debris or infection, myopia, sty, glaucoma)	Not seeing clearly	Ash Here and Now Cactus Indian Fig/Banyan Tree	Clay Italian Arum Water Lily
Fainting	'Get me out of here!'	Foxglove Heliconium	Peace Nostrum Isis Hyacinth
Fatigue	Struggle and conflict with the self 'Do I, don't I?' 'I don't want to do this but I don't know what else there is.'	Lamium	Heather Isis Lilac Seaside Centaury Velvet Bentgrass Water Lily
Fear	Inability to deal with fear is usually due to a dysfunctional base chakra	Heliconium Flamboyant Tree Silver Banksia Blackberry	Christ Ray Athena Summer Solstice Lammas
Feet	Can indicate our own perception of our body as in reflexology, or the means by which to move with stability	Hazel Silver Princess	Musk Orchid
Female cycle problems (heavy periods, irregular periods, fibroids)	Dislike of the feminine principle, due to fear, lack of confidence. Seeing the feminine as weak	Silver Princess Casuarina Flowers Silky Oak	Motherwort Spring Equinox
Food poisoning	Body's defences are down, allowing infiltration and attack by bacteria	Silver Banksia En Tears of Christ Blackberry	Lilac Sun Orchid Yarrow White
Fractures	Tired, worn out, asking for a break	Lemon	Water Moss Golden Rutilated Quartz
Frigidity	Dysfunctional beliefs in the sexual action, usually due to abuse, resulting in fear	Lemon Orange Passion Flower	Musk Orchid
Fungal infections (athlete's foot)	Living in the past and not moving forward	Hazel Green Alkanet	Heartsease Mary Hyacinth Blue

Symptom	Reason/Emotion (How you are now – where you want to be)	Flower Leader	Flower Helper
Gallstones	Life is bitter, resentment	Buddleia	Water Lily Sweet Flag Grass Purple Iris Alpine Bittercress Love in a Mist
Gastroenteritis	Unable to assimilate information	Mountain Ash Hazel	Imbolc
Glandular problems	Inertia. Your 'get-up-and-go' has gone!	Peace Nostrum Blackberry	Lilac Water Moss Athena
Gout	Control and anger	Iolite Hazel	Summer Solstice Demeter Common Wallflower
Gum problems (bleeding, gingivitis)	Indecision	Lamium	Water Moss Velvet Bentgrass Seaside Centaury Heather
Haemorrhoids	Fear of letting go, stuck for time	Blackberry	Olive Beltane
Hayfever	Denying the self as powerful, guilt	Judas Tree En Orange	Pine Heart to Heart
Headaches (migraine)	Critical and denying of self	Birch Mary	Venus Orchid Pine Heather
Hearing problems (tinnitus)	Not wanting to hear something	Apple Golden Wattle Foxglove	Clay Water Moss Italian Arum Shadow Cactus
– glue ear (*see Loss of balance*)			
Heart attack	A hardened, sad heart	Rose She-Oak Casuarina Flowers	Love in a Mist Couch Grass Heather
Heartburn (peptic ulcer, digestive problems)	Ultimately fear, withdrawing ourselves from painful situations	Buddleia Silver Banksia	Sweet Flag Grass Timothy Grass Shadow Cactus

SYMPTOM	REASON/EMOTION (How you are now – where you want to be)	FLOWER LEADER	FLOWER HELPER
Hepatitis	Anger, anger, anger and refusing to let go of it	Peace Nostrum Blackberry Passion Flower Mary Cedar Sunset	Star of Bethlehem Alpine Bittercress Fuchsia/Athena Marsh Helleborine Common Wallflower
Hernia	Straining to make a relationship work	Lemon Passion Flower	Motherwort Thistle Heart to Heart
Herpes (genital)	Sexual guilt	Judas Tree En Orange Lemon	Wormwood/Lammas Cyclamen/Athena
Hip problems	Stuck, can't move forward due to fear and/or lack of confidence	Casuarina Flowers Silky Oak	Rowan Citrine Grounding Opuntia Cactus Wych Elm Spring Equinox
Hodgkin's Disease/Lymphoma	Feeling you are not good enough, long-term childhood issues of not being loved and feeling worthless	Baobab	Rowan Couch Grass
Huntington's Disease	Trying to control, others and yourself – usually have controlling parent	St John's Wort (if appropriate)	Motherwort Heather Peace Nostrum Oak Blue Spirea
Hypoglycaemia (see Diabetes)			
Impotence	Perceived sexual pressures – can be mother-dominated. Retreating and closing down the heart	Lemon Orange Passion Flower	Motherwort Roseroot Snowdrop Demeter
Incontinence	Flooding of emotions. In later years – due to a build-up of undemonstrated emotions. After childbirth – keeping feelings and anxieties to yourself	Alder Wormwood/Lammas	Demeter Frangipani Love in a Mist
Indigestion	Anxiety, starting to close down the process of giving and receiving love	Buddleia Blackberry Alder	Love in a Mist Timothy Grass Shadow Cactus

Symptom	Reason/Emotion (How you are now – where you want to be)	Flower Leader	Flower Helper
Infertility	Fear of the future	Christ Ray Heliconium Ivy Lime (Linden) Stellaris	Heather Demeter

Inflammations and Infections

Inflammation is usually characterized by the following four symptoms: redness, heat, swelling and pain. Pain and Oedema have been listed separately below. Inflammation can be the result of infection (bacteria and virus infiltration) or trauma.

Symptom	Reason/Emotion	Flower Leader	Flower Helper
Inflammation and infections (systemic infections – flu, temperature – wound sepsis, sore throat)	Angry and incensed (*see individual symptoms*)	Peace Nostrum Blackberry	Lilac Imbolc
Insomnia	Too much going on, can't 'switch off' or feeling out of sync with cycles and circadian rhythms	Silver Princess Cedar Sunset	Lilac Pine Oak Peace Nostrum
Itchy skin problems	Wanting a different outcome, sadness, itching to change	Birch	Lilac Sand Rush Grass Water Moss
Jaw problems (TMJ– tempo-) romandibular joint	Wanting revenge	Aaron's Rod Peace Nostrum Strumpfia	Star of Bethlehem Venus Orchid
Kidney problems	Having felt like a failure, turning your disappointment and extreme critical views on yourself and others	Hawthorn Black Wattle	Thistle Maize Gardenia/Mary Citrine Scurvy Grass
Knee problems	Feeling superior to others, having an exacerbated sense of self	Strumpfia Ash Casuarina Flowers	Knotgrass Rowan Summer Solstice Sun Orchid European Spindle Tree

SYMPTOM	REASON/EMOTION (How you are now – where you want to be)	FLOWER LEADER	FLOWER HELPER
Leg problems	Legs take us forward in life and problems indicate a fear of moving on	Rivet Wheat *Anything for fear*	Mary Snowdrop Couch Grass Marsh Helleborine
Leukaemia	Blood is representative of your life force; when you have given up on life your life force is stagnant and has no life or vibrancy	Casuarina Flowers Passion Flower	Shakti Agrimony Citrine
Liver problems (jaundice, hepatitis)	Anger sits comfortably in the liver and ensures our validation of our own deceptions of truth	Bakul Tree Magnolia Centaurea	Water Lily Fuchsia/Athena Scolecite Ceanothus Common Wallflower
Loss of balance (inner ear infection, labyrinthitis)	Trying desperately to keep a balance in your life	Strumpfia Snow Gum Green Alkanet	Pine
Lung problems	Need to get something off your chest	Cedar Sunset	Heather
Lymphatic problems	Lack of love or happiness in your life, starting to give up	Flame Tree Magnolia	Olive CommonWallflower/ Demeter
ME (Myalgic Encephalomyelitis)	Living on chaos can cause a physical shutdown. Toxic adrenaline dependency for over-achieving personality. Fear of not being good enough, something to prove	Flamboyant Tree Blackberry Foxglove	Oriental Helleborine Couch Grass Sun Orchid Love in a Mist Thistle Rowan Star of Bethlehem
Menopause problems	Fear of the ageing process and the unknown	Christ Ray Bakul Tree	Demeter Rowan
Miscarriage/abortion	Fear of the unknown	Christ Ray Rivet Wheat	Birch Rowan
Mouth ulcers	What is stopping you with new ideas, eating away at your thoughts for the future?	Mandrake Blackberry	Water Moss Shakti

Symptom	Reason/Emotion (How you are now – where you want to be)	Flower Leader	Flower Helper
Multiple sclerosis	Extreme inflexibility and irritability due to fear, causing you to try to control all situations around you	Green Alkanet Ash Casuarina Flowers	Imbolc Orange Azalea Summer Solstice Water Lily Oak Rowan Wych Elm
Muscular problems	Muscles are tissues that move, problems represent an inability to go with the flow	Magnolia Ajuga/Peace Nostrum Alder Buddleia White Mangrove Lamium	Tobacco Plant/ Demeter Love in a Mist Grounding Opuntia Cactus
Nausea/morning sickness	Fear *Try visualizing breathing deep red into your perineum (or bottom if you find this easier), a little difficult when you're throwing up, but you have to breathe anyway, so focus on the colour red as you do	Buddleia Heliconium	Love in a Mist Musk Orchid
Neck problems (stiffness, tension, whiplash)	Having an inflexible attitude and approach to issues in your life	Passion Flower Ash Casuarina Flowers	Water Moss Knotgrass Rowan
Nerves	As our receivers and transmitters, any nerve problems indicate that your lines of communication are down	Primula/Peace Nostrum Cedar Sunset Lime (Linden) Wormwood Victorian Christmas Bush	Rowan Water Lily Frangipani Olive Quaking Grass Oak Golden Rutilated Quartz Star of Bethlehem
Nervous breakdown	Breakdown of communication to the self, overwhelmed	Baobab Magnolia Peace Nostrum Victorian Christmas Bush	Sun Orchid Frangipani Olive Golden Rutilated Quartz Star of Bethlehem
Numbness (palsy, paralysis)	Holding back: arms – love and communication legs – fear and protection facial – communication	Blackberry Foxglove	Verbena Shadow Cactus

Symptom	Reason/Emotion (How you are now – where you want to be)	Flower Leader	Flower Helper
Obesity	Fearful, needing protection	Red River Gum Bay Cedar	Thistle
Oedema/water retention	Trauma to emotions and physical trauma	En Soft Rush Grass	Scurvy Grass
Osteoporosis	Crumbling support (financial or family)	Lemon Flamboyant Tree	Sand Rush Grass Winter Solstice
Pain	Trapped energy – or stopping the flow of energy. See the appropriate body part – natural communication from the body is suffering: 'Hey, listen to me there's a problem in here'	Mountain Ash Wild Cherry Silver Banksia	Star of Bethlehem Alpine Bittercress
Panic attacks (palpitations, fainting, hyperventilation)	Frustration, addiction to chaos, 'I can't do this'	Victorian Christmas Bush Wild Cherry Lamium	Star of Bethlehem Wych Elm Scolecite Mandrake Hyacinth Blue
Parasitic infections	Giving away your power, letting others feed off you – getting sucked into someone else's game	Bay Cedar	Golden Rutilated Quartz Beltane
Premenstrual syndrome (PMS)	Dislike of the feminine principle, due to fear, lack of confidence	Silver Princess Casuarina Flowers Silky Oak Christ Ray	Motherwort Heather Rowan Spring Equinox

Protection

Fear and the need for protection are as fundamental as oxygen and food to our bodies. We have our own protective system set in place from day one – three energetic points that are essential for keeping our body protected and safe from attack: the base chakra and two points either side of the ears. The left ear is responsible for fight and the repair of the force field in physical terms, this point is linked with the immune system. The right ear is responsible for flight or impetus to escape from danger and this point is linked with the hormones, especially adrenaline. As long as these points work we have no need for extra protection from any other source, as our own innate force field is more than adequate to deal with anything from physical danger, to bugs in the air or psychic attack. It is only when any or all of these points become dysfunctional there is a problem. So how do they get broken or dysfunctional?

The process of bodily protection is primarily from the production of adrenaline, which helps you to retreat from danger or stand and fight (fight-or-flight response). The other aspect is the body's own repair and maintenance team: the internal protection from the immune system and its response to internal and external intruders. When the body falls into disrepair the cross energy from these two points (on either side of the ears) ceases to function properly and the force field that is usually apparent also no longer functions. The cross energy has the ability to move or flip, and can flip from positive to negative very easily. When it is positive it repels and when in a negative mode it loses its ability to repel and becomes sticky.

We all need to feel protected – either an inner sense of security or, if we don't have this due to abuse or other trauma, we try to find it elsewhere: our job, house, mortgage, friends, finances. So we fall into fear and this starts the cycle of fear, loss, protection, control. Others who need more protection are empaths – sensitive individuals who pick up on others' emotions just by being in their energy field. These people can get lost in the feelings they experience and assume they are their own and this can cause disaster as they try to find a reason for the anger, sadness or whatever. Even if you are not supersensitive you can be affected by other people's energies when in close proximity to their aura, or energy field. Trains, buses, tube trains, and supermarkets are the hot spots to avoid – easy if you don't eat or work, and stay home like a hermit, very hungry! I don't eat meat but have been known to get to the checkout of the supermarket with a couple of steaks that someone else wanted!

Many physical symptoms have their origins in fear. There are many roads to and from fear, from motorways to dirt tracks, with each having their own set of nuances. By using the flower essence profiles and reading about that chapter's unique angle you will be able to make some inroads for your own protection.

Symptom	Reason/Emotion (How you are now – where you want to be)	Flower Leader	Flower Helper
Protection	Insecurity, fear	Tears of Christ Silver Banksia Yew Bay Cedar	Iolite Grounding Opuntia Cactus Quaking Grass Sun Orchid
Psychiatric problems (insanity, depression, self-esteem issues)	Retreating from reality, inability to cope with family issues	Spider Lily Baobab	Demeter Ceanothus Citrine

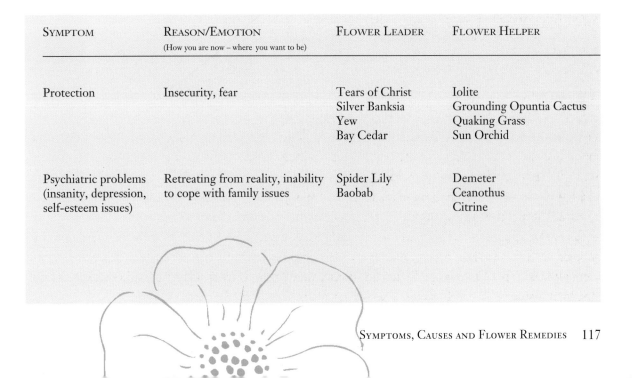

Symptom	Reason/Emotion (How you are now – where you want to be)	Flower Leader	Flower Helper
Rashes (hives, urticaria)	Irritation	Birch	Holly Winter Solstice Orange Azalea Purple Toadflax
Respiratory (respiratory ailments, colds and flu, coughs, bronchitis)	A need to get something off your chest	Lamium Cedar Sunset Snowdrop	Cedar Couch Grass Demeter Heather
Rheumatism	Having a victim mentality – 'poor me' syndrome. Lack of love, resentment	Tears of Christ Lemon Snow Gum Soft Rush Grass	Frangipani Alpine Bittercress Knotgrass Maize Sand Rush Grass
Scar tissue	Blame – reminder of trauma, needing to let go and heal	Orange	Water Moss
Sciatica	Denying the self of abundance	Flame Tree	Stargazer lily Golden Rutilated Quartz Grounding Opuntia Cactus Clay Demeter
Seizures	Get me out of here	Victorian Christmas Bush	Purple Toadflax
Self-inflicted wounds	Looking for attention or needing to feel	Here and Now Cactus	Sun Orchid
Sexually transmitted diseases (gonorrhoea, genital herpes, VD, chlamydia)	Guilt	Orange Judas Tree En	Christ Ray Rowan
Shingles	Oversensitive	Bay Cedar White Mangrove	Clay Geranium Lilac

Shock and Trauma

Most, if not all, symptoms you experience are the direct and indirect result of a shock or trauma, so it is imperative that you deal with this first and foremost. If you visit any conventional medical specialist, whether your own GP or Casualty, the first thing they will assess is the amount of shock or trauma: make sure you are breathing and your heart is beating and assess and treat any abnormalities. Your energy system is no different: energy flows from the planet and universe into your energy field and is synchronized with your breathing, so it follows that any disruption to this is going to have an effect on the mechanics of your body. Likewise, your body's force field, its own protection system in the form of cross energy, is synchronized with your heartbeat. These are always the first lines of defence to be compromised. Shock and trauma, if not dealt with emotionally, can linger in your body many years after the event and pop up to affect you when you least expect it. If you don't have any of the symptoms listed and want to try an essence, a good place to start is to negate any effects of shock to your emotional body by taking one of the essences listed below.

Symptom	Reason/Emotion (How you are now – where you want to be)	Flower Leader	Flower Helper
Shock and trauma	Disbelief	Centaurea En Tears of Christ Rose She-Oak Baobab Lemon Silver Banksia	Judas Tree Star of Bethlehem Thistle Demeter Love in a Mist Marsh Helleborine
Shoulder problems	Overburdened by responsibility and not voicing your own needs	Peace Nostrum Blue Gum Passion Flower	Venus Orchid Maize Common Wallflower Beltane
Sickness and vomiting (morning sickness, travel sickness)	Fear, no control of the situation	Heliconium Silver Princess	Sweet Flag Grass Love in a Mist
Sinusitis	Irritation to sensory information	Strumpfia Hazel Here and Now Cactus Horsetail She-Oak Ash Soft Rush Grass	Orange Azalea Purple Toadflax Venus Orchid Frangipani Holly
Skeletal problems	Resentment affecting the structure of your life	Lemon Lime (Linden) Flame Tree Green Alkanet Wormwood	Purple Iris/Hathor Darnel Grass

Skin Problems

As humans we suffer the greatest of human characteristics – emotion. Sometimes, due to the way you are raised by your parents, you emulate their reactions. If they are not responsive and tactile you follow their lead and become aloof. You may try to keep the peace and not show feelings because you don't want to hurt or be hurt. Just because emotions aren't showing, it doesn't mean they aren't there: bubbling away underneath is the unexpressed fear and sadness. Take my word for it – it has to come out one way or another. The skin is the largest organ your body has, so your body may use it to release the emotions that you are unable to release willingly. As soon as you take control and agree to let these emotions out, the skin will cease to be the outlet.

SYMPTOM	REASON/EMOTION (How you are now – where you want to be)	FLOWER LEADER	FLOWER HELPER
Skin problems (acne, blemishes, eczema, psoriasis, rashes)	Inappropriate emotional release	Lime (*either or both*) Orange Birch Lemon Passion Flower Silver Princess	Holly Oak Lilac Hathor Motherwort Winter Solstice Heartsease Peace Nostrum Frangipani
Snoring	Challenges with changing cycles and a need for protection	Bakul Tree Cedar Sunset	Demeter Purple Toadflax
Sore throat	Unable to speak out about angry thoughts	Black Wattle Ajuga	Scurvy Grass Ceanothus/Betony
Speech problems (stutter, developmental problems)	Insecure, frightened, the eternal peace keeper	Peace Nostrum Indian Fig/Banyan Tree	Thistle Heather
Sprains	Victim of fear, wanting to stay in the back seat	Buddleia St John's Wort Flamboyant Tree Heliconium	Yarrow/Mary Thistle Geranium
Stiff joints	For remaining flexible, for a controlling personality (*see also Aches and pains*)	Casuarina Flowers	Knotgrass Rowan
Stomach (ulcers, indigestion)	Resistance to change, wanting life to stay the same. 'I'm right, you're wrong'	Buddleia Alder Blackberry	Water Lily Agrimony Alpine Bittercress Knotgrass Timothy Grass Sweet Flag Grass

Symptom	Reason/Emotion (How you are now – where you want to be)	Flower Leader	Flower Helper
Stress	Overburdened	Lime (*either or both*) Victorian Xmas Bush Lamium Alder Oriental Hellebore	Venus Orchid Frangipani Holly Pine Demeter
Stroke (CVA)	Will not change, refusal to have a heart-to-heart exchange, avoidance	Christ Ray Lamium Foxglove	Thistle Golden Rutilated Quartz Water Moss Peace Nostrum Heart to Heart Darnel Grass Fuchsia/Athena Hellebore/Demeter
Suicidal tendencies	End of the road, cannot or will not see another way forward	Spider Lily Victorian Christmas Bush Magnolia	Agrimony Darnel Grass Olive
Swollen glands	Procrastination and putting off making decisions	Magnolia Lamium Mountain Ash Rivet Wheat	Dianthus/Isis Lilac
Teeth	Memories and indecision about their truth or illusion	Apple Rivet Wheat	Clay Christmas Cactus Water Moss
Testicular problems	Issues relating to one's masculinity	St John's Wort Strumpfia	Grounding Opuntia Cactus Holly
Thrush	Questioning the decisions in life, wishy-washy	Magnolia Lamium Blackberry	Seaside Centaury Velvet Bentgrass Water Lily Heather
Thyroid problems (hyperthyroidism, hypothyroidism)	'Pity party' time – feeling sorry for yourself all the time: 'It's not fair – I never get to do what I want to do.' Humiliation, reactive personality – metabolic issue	Tears of Christ Passion Flower	Water Moss Ceanothus/Isis Citrine
Tinnitus (*see Hearing problems*)		Strumpfia	Shadow Cactus

Symptom	Reason/Emotion (How you are now – where you want to be)	Flower Leader	Flower Helper
Tonsillitis (quinsy, peritonsillar abscess)	Suppressed communication – fear of reprisals	Ajuga/Peace Nostrum Indian Fig/Banyan Tree Black Wattle	Water Moss Forget-Me-Not Olive Thistle Lilac
Tuberculosis	Overcome with negativity (see also appropriate place in body)	Hawthorn Orange Silver Banksia Rock Jasmine/Peace Nostrum	Geranium Marsh Helleborine Holly
Tumours	Refusal to let hurt and pain go	Blackberry Christ Ray Rock Jasmine/Peace Nostrum Buddleia	Alpine Bittercess Heartsease Love in a Mist
Urinary infections	Angry and 'peed off'	Tears of Christ Ajuga/Peace Nostrum	Rowan Maize Verbena
Urticaria (hives) (*See Rashes*)			
Uterine problems	Creativity and its ease or 'dis-ease'	Casuarina Flowers Silver Princess	Stargazer Lily Citrine Beltane Lammas Cyclamen
Vaginitis/Bartholin's cyst	Partner and sexual relationship issues	Lemon Passion Flower Orange Lemon	Heartsease Thistle Water Moss
Varicose veins	Stagnant puddle? Being in a situation you find unbearable	Aaron's Rod Magnolia Flame Tree Peace Nostrum	Jasmine White Love in a Mist Grounding Opuntia Cactus Agrimony
Vertigo (dizziness)	Seeing a different reality to what you believe	Centaurea Lime (*either*) Strumpfia	Scolecite Water Lily

SYMPTOM	REASON/EMOTION (How you are now – where you want to be)	FLOWER LEADER	FLOWER HELPER
Viral infections (AIDS, chickenpox, cytomegalovirus (CMV))	Not liking oneself. Extreme self-esteem and confidence, usually because the second chakra overcompensates for a dysfunctional base chakra	Silver Princess Silky Oak Heliconium	Samhain Timothy Grass Ceanothus/Isis
Vitiligo	Feeling different to everyone else, not fitting in (See also fFowers for confidence)	Green Alkanet Silky Oak	Tobacco Plant/ Demeter
Vomiting (see Nausea, Fear)			
Warts/verrucae (see Viral infections)	Self-esteem issues	Silver Princess Casuarina Flowers	Wych Elm Frangipani
Wisdom teeth	Problems with wisdom teeth are usually because of lack of space, hemmed in	Lemon Casuarina Flowers	Past Life Orchid Cedar Scolecite
Yeast infections (candida, thrush)	'I don't exist, everyone else comes first', allowing yourself to be invaded	Flamboyant Tree Cedar Sunset	Blue Spiraea Heartsease Winter Solstice Gaia

Working with Children

As I've said many times, essences are completely safe for anyone to take, so when you give these wonderful droplets to your most precious offspring you can be safe in the knowledge that you are not harming them in any way, shape or form. Parents often ask: 'Will they work for my child? Don't you have to believe in the medicine for it to work?' The answer is definitely yes, they will work, and more importantly, you don't have to believe in their efficacy for the wonders of essences to work their magic on you. Having said that, you can reduce their ability to get through by putting up a resistance. Children, however, don't have this on their agenda – why would they? Their only concern is to be happy and fulfilled.

Children are often upset because of the group energy being circulated at home. In my practice I am continually treating patients with serious communication, relationship and sexual issues because of incidents that happened in their childhood. No doubt you also have concerns that could be traced back to how you felt during your formative years, so think hard about how your child is feeling when you next let rip at someone or something in the home. Just recently a five-year-old was trying to put his shoes in a cupboard and was heard to say, 'Bloody shoes, bloody shoes'. When asked why he was using such language he replied to his mother, 'I'm angry and you say bloody when you are angry'.

Feeding difficulties, whether with babies or toddlers, are usually helped by mum and dad sorting out a couple of essences for themselves first, precisely for this reason. If your children are taking essences then you should be also, just to be on the safe side. Summer Solstice Goddess and Venus Orchid are both wonderful for parent support.

How do you choose an essence for a child? If they can talk, you can obviously ask a few pertinent questions, but this doesn't help you if you are the worried parent of a baby, trying to work out why it is upset. Intuits™ can be done, by you, by the carer, for your child, or by the child itself as long as he/she can count to ten. Alternatively I have suggested just a few scenarios that come up for children below.

Peace of Mind

One cannot overdose on essences. Flower essences are primarily vibrational in nature, which means that they are non-toxic and you can't take too much, unless you drink a huge quantity and are affected by the alcohol used as a preservative. It's an interesting element of taking your essence that a 15ml bottle will usually last two weeks, give or take a dose. Ever since I can remember I have taken my essence conscientiously every day, twice a day, dosing the prescribed amount of drops – but sometimes the bottle lasts one week and sometimes three, how I have no idea. My sources tell me that we instinctively know if we don't want to take it and so we reduce the amount unconsciously. On the other side of the coin, we can finish it off quicker than blinking, obviously needing it more than has been prescribed.

Babies and smaller children have you to give them the dose. I prepare essences for children in vegetable glycerine – not alcohol – and they love the taste. They can be taken neat from the dropper or given in a little water if preferred. Older children love the responsibility of taking their own essence and once taught will be meticulous with self-administration. My own boys have grown up taking 'fairy drops' – although now that they are aged 16 and 17, the fairy has well and truly been dropped. They even suggest essences for their friends.

On the children's chart the first column shows the problem, the second a possible emotional cause, the third recommended Leaders, the next a selection of Helpers, and the last the ideal outcome. As mentioned before, it is impossible for me to specify an exact Helper without knowing details of the child and the problem, so either you or your child can use the Intuits™ system to choose one for yourself – see page 141 for instructions.

Essences for Children

Symptom	Possible Emotional Cause	Leader	Helper	Outcome
Asthma	Fear of life, stifled	Flamboyant Tree En Green Alkanet	Star of Bethlehem Frangipani Golden Rutilated Quartz Motherwort	Focused, new-found sense of freedom
Bedwetting	Usually due to fear – parents need to be aware of their own impact on the fearful child	St John's Wort Heliconium	Frangipani Water Lily Geranium Motherwort	Dry bed for a start and a more confident child
Behaviour (ADHD, dyslexia, dyspraxia, etc)	Frustration, feeling insecure (*see Note on page 127*)	Lamium En Flamboyant Tree Peace Nostrum	Love in a Mist Geranium Purple Toadflax Sun Rose Olive	Ease of being who they are – beautiful
Birth trauma	New life can be very frightening for the newborn. Lovely to add to the bath water	En Baobab Birch	Motherwort Star of Bethlehem Forget-Me-Not Vibernum Ceanothus	Settled baby
Being bullied	Allowing yourself to be bullied usually indicates fear and lack of self-esteem	Iolite St John's Wort Magnolia	Sun Rose Stargazer Lily	Assertive and unafraid
Croup	Discontent in the home situation, unfavourable group energy causing stress	Peace Nostrum (Black) Lime (Linden) Bay Cedar	Heather Holly Lamium Citrine	Feeling of space allows them to open up, breathe easier (in meta physical sense)
Crying (excessive)	Emotional release	Peace Nostrum Blue Gum Foxglove	Iolite Lilac Scolecite	Allows the child to verbalize their sadness and pain and move on

Symptom	Possible Emotional Cause	Leader	Helper	Outcome
Eczema	Inappropriate emotional release (*see Skin problems in Essences for Adults*)			
Hyperactivity	Needing to feel secure	Spider Lily Flamboyant Tree Giant Honey Myrtle Oriental Hellebore	Here And Now Cactus Orange Azalea	Calms and centres
Nail biting	Unable to communicate with parents, frustration	Peace Nostrum Aaron's Rod Flame Tree	Purple Iris Geranium Agrimony	No bitten nails and less anxious
Nosebleeds	Desperate for love and attention	Horsetail She-Oak White Mangrove Viper's Bugloss	Alpine Bittercress Sun Orchid Geranium Wormwood	Feeling nurtured within
Runny nose	A form of crying, or a cry for help	Ajuga Blackberry	Ceanothus/ Isis Orange Azalea Vibernum Frangipani	Runny noses limited to colds
Silence (as bad as rowing)	Withdrawing, what's the point?	Cedar Sunset Spider Lily Iolite	Ceanothus/ Isis Tobacco Plant	Interaction with the family without the need for loneliness
Studying/exams	Unable to focus	Magnolia Hazel	Imbolc Past Life Orchid	Determined and getting on with life
Tantrums	Frustration at not being able to communicate	Foxglove Wild Cherry Pipil Tzin-Tzintli	Holly Love in a Mist Lilac	Calm shopping trips, happy children, happy mum
Thumb sucking, dummies, security blanket	Needing security	Flame Tree Heliconium Victorian Christmas Bush	Love in a Mist Stargazer Lily	Cuddles and hugs instead

Note

This section on children would not be complete without mention of the difficulties that are experienced by a child after a diagnosis of one of the various developmental issues: ADD, ADHD, Dyslexia, Dyspraxia, Autism, Asperger's Syndrome, Tourette's Syndrome. All these children, without exception, are very sensitive individuals. Understandably they are very frustrated at their apparent lack of ability to communicate effectively, and this inevitably gives way to low self-esteem and lack of confidence. As my son was diagnosed with ADHD when he was two years old, I have experienced first-hand the challenges to him and to me, as his mother – not to mention the problems that come up with kindergarten, sports and schoolteachers. I have told you how I first came to learn about essences and how my instruction to this day still comes from my inner tuition. I 'know' from experience and research that this spectrum of dis-orders is an energetic programming dysfunction. My understanding of this is quite simple.

Imagine your spirit or soul: the sum total of your experiences in this life and others before. Now imagine your physical body – the coat you have been given to perform your tasks on this planet. The membrane in between is the interface, where communication takes place between these two bodies. My belief is that with these children the spirit or soul operates on the equivalent of Windows XP and the body works on Windows 95 – a bit of a problem without the programming software to convert the information received and sent. I believe that the interface is dysfunctional – putting my nurse's hat on, that would equate to the brain. Over the past eight years, I have been making and researching essences to help this dysfunction. This treatment has developed from knowledge of the anatomy of our energy – and both my own experience and that of others who have gone though the therapy – bears it out. For parents of these – and other – very special children, my only suggestion is to take essences yourself to help you through this challenging period, and to enable you to help the child deal with the frustration and self-esteem issues for which they need support. Don't for one moment think they do not want to be here – they do, and they have a huge task changing our beliefs on how we view society and our small-minded attitudes as to what is 'normal'.

Case Study

One of my patients – I'll call her Sue – has two autistic children. Her own healing from the childhood abuse she suffered has been profound, helped by the teaching of her adorable little girls. After a very physically and sexually abusive childhood, her mother sent Sue away to a children's home time and time again. All she wanted was for her mother to love her, but over the years Sue became very angry and abusive herself and found that if she bullied and hit out, she could get exactly what she wanted. That was until her own children came along. Of course, bullying didn't get her anywhere, shouting didn't cut it either, and she became more angry with her apparent lack of control. With her old ways not working at all she had to try another way and, hey presto, some changes. As she continued to take essences, have Bodylink energy therapy and talk through her own issues, she could see that love, kindness and working with her children rather than against them produced much more favourable results. She loves these little darlings more than life itself and couldn't hurt one hair of their curly blond hair. Far from angry, she is now their closest ally and they respond to her with love. The children have responded really well to the essences, are now playing with each other, accept other carers, listen to stories and recently, out of the blue, told her that they love her.

Essences for Animals

Animals, like children, respond extremely well to essences, but of course the challenge is finding the perfect essence or mixture to benefit your pet. Animals, as we all know, can communicate with their owners – maybe not verbally, but every owner knows their pet's basic needs. What can appear to be an aggressive, controlling animal can in reality be a pet that is fearful and just needs a hug, if only he or she will let you. Intuits™ for animals is perfect for finding out what your pet really needs; they are easily chosen by the owner, with amazing success, and give the opportunity to readjust your pet's emotions.

I can't emphasize enough the importance of communicating with your pet. Talk to it, tell it that you are going to take it to the vet for whatever cause, or that you want to understand why it is urinating in the house. Use a soft tone and understanding attitude – shouting and being aggressive will only make the situation worse. If you are angry, you may need an essence also.

Animals are fabulous teachers; they are able to help us heal and feel safe, loved, cared for and nurtured. All they ask in return is to be fed, watered and loved back. So how do they teach us? Remember, they are an integral part of your household and, as such, sense the combined energy or 'feel' of the house. In reality they show us what is happening. A divorce or break-up can send some pets into crisis because of the tension. A new baby on the scene often throws up jealousy, when the husband/father shows the same tendency. For those of you familiar with the television show *The Osbornes*, what did their dogs do when there was strife, anger and shouting in the house? They turned the house into a litter tray whenever the tone of the house became a little stressed.

It's important to remember that if the emotional problem persists you may want to also try one of the following as well:

ANIMAL HEALING – Using hands, to impart energy to the animal for balance, health and reassurance.
ANIMAL COMMUNICATOR – Using the ability to communicate with animals through the art of telepathy.
TELLINGTON TOUCH – Developed by Linda Tellington-Jones, this method can improve behavioural, physical, health and performance issues. It can also help you, the owner, communicate with your animal by working together with the trainer.

Obviously if your pet needs physical attention, your vet should always be your first port of call, but pets also need emotional support and that's where the essences come into their own.

Dosing

I usually make essences for animals in vegetable glycerine, a little sweet but much better than alcohol. My own cat loves them and will let me put them straight into her mouth. If you do this also you will need to sterilize the dropper in boiling water after each dose to eliminate the possibility of bacteria growing in the bottle between doses. Another way of dosing is to add the essence to food but if you have more than one animal make sure that the animal you are treating eats its own food. If they like to share, just place the drops on a small amount of food for the animal having treatment and once the food had been eaten, give the remainder of the meal. It doesn't matter if the other animal gets the dose, but this does mean that the animal needing it only gets a fraction.

The analysis of the results from Intuits™ for animals is very interesting. It would seem that cats and dogs are very different in their approach to life emotionally. After all, we all know that they behave differently, so why should they not have different emotions? The most commonly chosen essence for cats is Heliconium, for fear. This essence does not appear on the list for dogs except in two instances where the dog vomited continuously on car journeys. The top essence for dogs is Seaside Centaury, for clarity. Again we have the same picture, with only two instances of the essence ever having been chosen for cats, where they were both extremely stressed by the introduction of another animal into the household. We have here opposite sides of the spectrum, Heliconium for the base chakra and Seaside Centaury for the crown chakra. I have only mentioned essences here that have been chosen for animals, out of the list of over 150 in the book.

It would seem that most problems that occur with cats are a temporary blip in their intuition and are due to the trials and tribulations of being a physical creature. These animals are truly spiritual beings having a physical experience, and can stay on top of their emotions most of the time. If they don't like a situation, they move on and find a new home. They suffer mostly from physical complaints associated with cleansing and the release of toxic matter, as they are also clearing our emotions most of the time. Think of them as 'emotional vacuum cleaners', which also get blocked sometimes. As very sensitive beings they are prone to being territorial and like their own space, since most of their time is spent in deep meditation – not asleep. Most animal welfare societies and vets support spaying or neutering animals for many reasons, but let's look at the emotional aspect. The emotional behaviour of the animal is altered by this procedure, making them less likely to fight and spray their territory and, interestingly enough, eliminating the possibility of uterine, breast, ovarian and testicular cancer. Not that I am advocating this for one minute, but I wonder if this would work on humans? However, since cats are here to help us, are we not taking that ability away from them? A question indeed. When they exhibit disgusting behaviour they are perhaps only reflecting their carer's own issues and are trying desperately to show you the unrest at home. Even after the animal has been altered they do at times still show the same behaviour patterns. They certainly have their work cut out with us. They want love and want to teach you how to love. The next time you fight, argue, or get jealous, think of the cats.

Essences for Cats

Symptom	Possible Cause	Leader	Helper	Possible Outcome
Aggressive (fighting with other animals)	This is my space, fighting for own identity	Heliconium Snowdrop	Citrine Seaside Centaury Thistle	I'm cool, do you want to be friends?
Biting	– if the animal bites you, telling you to look at yourself – if biting another animal, is it saying you and your partner are hurting each other?	Heliconium Snowdrop	Holly Purple Iris/Hathor Seaside Centaury	Okay I'll find another way, do you want a cuddle?
Car/Travel sickness	Fear	Heliconium Passion Flower	Couch Grass Golden Rutilated Quartz	Wake me up when we're there

Symptom	Possible Cause	Leader	Helper	Possible Outcome
Clinging	Wanting to be loved, helping you to show love	Victorian Christmas Bush Passion Flower	Oak Stargazer Lily	I'm here when you're ready
Death of loved one (loneliness)	Grief at the loss of a friend	Victorian Christmas Bush Passion Flower	Crocus/Hathor Oak/Heart to Heart	I miss my friend but I'm okay
Fearful	Help me here, I need some compassion	Heliconium Red River Gum	Seaside Centaury Thistle	Chilled
Fireworks/loud noises	Fear and shock. Is this a memory of another previous trauma?	Heliconium Silverband	Pine Oak Golden Rutilated Quartz	Mmm, what noise?
Health issues (Support for animals)	(See Essences for adults)	Snowdrop	Couch Grass Clay	I know I'm being looked after
In season	Not again. Do you, her owner, also have PMT?	Lemon Passion Flower	Motherwort	What PMT? I'm great
Neutered/spayed	Confused – how would you feel?	Passion Flower	Crocus/ Hathor Couch Grass	Oh well, life goes on
New baby/animal	Alone, feeling abandoned	Lemon Victorian Christmas Bush	Seaside Centaury Motherwort Thistle Citrine	Another friend to play with/do you want love too?
Post-op recovery	Stress, disorientation	Snowdrop Lemon	Citrine Couch Grass Clay African Violet	Let's get on with it
Pregnancy	Loved up. Oooops!	Snowdrop Heart to Heart	Couch Grass Motherwort	Happy, contented
Relocation, holiday, house sit/cattery	Confused, excited. Territorial issues	Heliconium Red River Gum Victorian Xmas Bush	Crocus/Hathor Stargazer Lily	Will you be better than the last one? Let's try
Toilet habits	The animal is trying to tell you something important and the owner needs to be understanding	Passion Flower	Pine Golden Rutilated Quartz Stargazer Lily	I'm not 'peed' with you and I'm not going to poo on my own doorstep

Dogs

Man's best friend – why? It's been said that 'dogs have owners and cats have staff' – ain't that the truth? We've been talking about cats and how they are spiritual beings trying to teach us about ourselves – like most teachers they press our buttons. Sometimes we feel uncomfortable in their presence, as if they can see right through us. Whereas dogs are a different kettle of fish – they love us no matter what; they are more human than some humans and they give us a very long lead to hang ourselves with. The 'dog's way' is 'never mind, give it another go, you'll get it right eventually', whereas the cat gets impatient and wants to show us right here and now it's not the right thing to do. So is it any wonder they fight between themselves? They are coming from the opposite ends of the spectrum.

A dog is your companion everywhere, walking to the park, going for rides in the car, going on holiday – playing in the sand, fetching sticks, playing football and leading us by the hand when we can't see for ourselves. They laugh at us and themselves, whereas a cat is never wrong. And that's why we like dogs so much. If the truth were known we're all striving to be cats but we can relate to dogs easily because we're on the same path. We are here to show each other compassion and unconditional love. Personally, I think cats used to be dogs.

Rather like cats, dogs can and will reflect their owner's behaviour. If you are aggressive, the dog most certainly will be. You only have to look at the breed of dog to see the reflection of the owner. A study compiled by researchers from the University of California in San Diego showed that people consistently choose purebred dogs that resemble them, but are not so fussy when it comes to choosing a mongrel. I always thought that Bill Sykes's dog Bull's Eye – an English bull terrier – in *Oliver Twist* was a perfect match. The dog of an aggressive owner will take any amount of beating the owner cares to give, being loyal to the end, but it will display those aggressive characteristics of the owner to others. Now where have I seen that before? Children and their parents! So if we are looking for the emotional cause of a dog's behaviour we must not forget how the owner can impact on the pooch.

As I finished this last paragraph, an email came into my in-box with this story:

A farmer had some puppies he needed to sell so he painted a sign advertising the four pups and set about nailing it to a post on the edge of his yard. As he was driving the last nail into the post, he felt a tug on his overalls and he looked down into the eyes of a little boy. 'Mister,' he said, 'I want to buy one of your puppies.' 'Well,' said the farmer, as he rubbed the sweat off the back of his neck, 'These puppies come from fine parents and cost a good deal of money.' The boy dropped his head for a moment. Then reaching deep into his pocket, he pulled out a handful of change and held it up to the farmer. 'I've got 39 cents. Is that enough to take a look?' 'Sure,' said the farmer. And with that he let out a whistle. 'Here, Dolly!' he called. Out from the doghouse and down the ramp ran Dolly followed by four little balls of fur. The little boy pressed his face against the chain link fence and his eyes danced with delight. As the dogs made their way to the fence, he noticed something else stirring inside the doghouse. Slowly another little ball appeared, this one noticeably smaller. Down the ramp it slid. Then in a somewhat awkward manner, the pup began hobbling toward the others, doing its best to catch up.

'I want that one,' the boy said, pointing to the runt. The farmer knelt down at his side and said, 'Son, you don't want that puppy. He will never be able to run and play with you like these other dogs would.' With that the boy stepped back from the fence, reached down, and began rolling up one leg of his trousers. In doing so he revealed a steel brace running down both sides of his leg, attaching itself to a specially made shoe. Looking back up at the farmer, he said, 'You see, I don't run too well myself, and he will need someone who understands.' The farmer reached down and picked up the pup. Holding it carefully he handed it to the child. 'How much?' asked the boy. 'No charge,' answered the farmer, 'there's no charge for love.'

So the dog can be seen as another form of human being, but has compassion and unconditional love and affection simply oozing out of its pores as long as you let it.

Many symptoms that dogs exhibit can be purely from lack of socialization. They don't know how to be with other dogs, other humans and other animals. As they are like humans, we have to teach them the rules. Most dogs are taken away from their mothers at an early age and now have us as their teachers, so don't stop at toilet training – go the whole way. Puppy school is kindergarten for dogs.

Essences for Dogs

Symptom	Possible Cause	Leader	Helper	Possible Outcome
Aggressive – fighting with other animals	Aggression and ego. This is my space, fighting for own identity No experience of socialization	St John's Wort Bakul Tree Bay Cedar	Seaside Centaury Ash Casuarina Flowers European Spindle Tree Holly	I'm cool, do you want to be friends?
Biting	Fear	St John's Wort Birch Cedar Sunset	Blue Spirea Holly Common Wallflower European Spindle Tree	Okay, I will find another way, do you want to play?

Symptom	Possible Cause	Leader	Helper	Possible Outcome
Car sickness	Fear	Heliconium Buddleia Green Alakanet En	Seaside Centaury Holly Oak Geranium	Wake me up when we're there
Clinging, pining	Wanting to be loved, helping you to show love, insecurity, unconditional mothering issues	Ivy Fig Horsetail She-Oak Magnolia	Seaside Centaury Alpine Bittercress Christmas Cactus Motherwort	I'm here when you're ready
Death of loved one (loneliness)	Grief at the loss of a friend	Green Alkanet Rose She-Oak Magnolia	Seaside Centaury Geranium Frangipani	I miss my friend but I'm okay
Fearful	Help me here, I need some security	Rose She-Oak Victorian Christmas Bush Red River Gum	Orange Azalea Blue Iris Love in a Mist	Chilled
Fireworks/loud noises	Fear and shock. Is this a memory of another previous trauma?	En St John's Wort Hazel Victorian Christmas Bush	Blue Iris Geranium Christmas Cactus Wormwood Star of Bethlehem	Mmmm, what noise
Health issues (support for animals)	(See Elements for adults)	Hazel Wild Cherry Snow Gum	Oriental Hellebore Frangipani	I know I'm being looked after
In season	Not again. Do you, her owner, also have PMT?	Orange Rose She-Oak Silver Princess	Motherwort Frangipani Seaside Centaury	What PMT? I'm great
Neutered/spayed	Angry, confused – how would you feel?	Lamium Green Alkanet En Victorian Christmas Bush	Seaside Centaury Betony Wormwood Olive Wych Elm	Oh well, life goes on
New baby/animal	Jealous, feeling abandoned, insecurity	St John's Wort Blue Gum Ivy Lamium	Darnel Grass Lady's Smock Lilac Olive	Another friend to play with, do you want love too?

Symptom	Possible Cause	Leader	Helper	Possible Outcome
Post-op recovery	Stress, disorientation	Hazel Wild Cherry Rose She-Oak	Seaside Centaury Betony Wormwood Star of Bethlehem	Let's get on with it
Pregnancy	Loved up. Oooops!	Green Alkanet Giant Honey Myrtle	Motherwort Stargazer Lily Past Life Orchid	Happy, contented
Relocation, holiday, house sit/kennels	Confused, excited, fearful, needing stability	Hazel St John's Wort Green Alkanet	Mexican Tarragon Orange Azalea	Are you going to be better than the last one? Let's try
Toilet habits	Embarrassed and now quite fearful	Flamboyant Tree Flame Tree Lemon Red River Gum	Jasmine White Wormwood Love in a Mist	I'm not peed with you and I'm not going to poo on my own doorstep.

An interesting difference with cats and dogs concerning the 'accidents' they have at home is that the cat is trying to tell you something; the dog on the other hand simply can't hold it any longer and just has to go. Being very embarrassed at its little accident, the dog will shy away and be very apologetic, whereas the cat will show indifference.

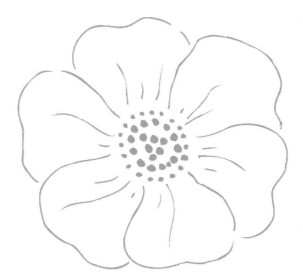

A Final Note

I don't have all the answers. In fact, in the grand scheme of things, I don't have many answers at all. Yet I do know that I understand and realize the importance of energy in our physical makeup and how it reacts with the matter that makes up the universe. We are but scratches on the scratch; change which will ultimately make a difference to our world can only begin with you, that tiny scratch. The more I learn, the more I realize what I don't know, and this keeps me yearning for more and more information. Every day is another opportunity to learn and put that knowledge to the test. I hope that this book creates a longing, a hunger that will not be satisfied, to know more. I asked at the start of my journey, 'Why me, I'm just a normal mum?' The reply came very loud and clear, 'That's exactly why.' I have questioned this response too many times since to count, and it never changes – maybe if I continually take my Osteospermum (South African Daisy) essence, I'll stop asking.

My hope is that this book lays the foundation for more questions from sources with the expertise to answer more probing questions. During this journey I've explained to every one of my clients what, where, and how, and have encouraged them to also question their responses and results. My clients include disabled children, dentists, doctors, scientists, nurses, businessmen and women, builders, taxi drivers, housewives, policemen, musicians, lawyers, teachers, retired pensioners, artists and babies and though the youngest was three months old and the oldest 82 years, every one of them moved on – no one ever went back to where they were before they started their journey.

Please question, but don't discount. At whatever point you join this journey and whatever your level of understanding, you can always move on from where you are now. At every resting point, question, be as cynical as you wish but leave your blinkers at home. Be receptive to accept, keep an open mind, and await the miracle of growth.

Thank you.

Combined Flower Essences

Combined essences comprise two or more flower essences. Issues that each essence can help with and sources are listed below.

Peace Nostrum
Flower essences: Ajuga, Lady's Smock, Marsh Marigold, Rock Jasmine, Yellow Primula
Key issues: Compassion, awareness
Recommended source: Bodylink Essences

Heart To Heart
Flower essences: Holly, Oak, Pine, Hailstones
Key issue: Finishing contracts
Recommended source: Bodylink Essences

Gaia – The Preserver
Flower essences: Heartsease, Hyssop, Myrtle
Key issues: Restoration; confidence
Recommended source: Gaia Essences

Isis – Divine Understanding
Flower essences: Ceanothus, Dianthus
Key issues: Connection with mind, body and spirit
Recommended source: Gaia Essences

Shakti – Sacred Energy
Flower essences: Impatiens, Marigold, Wallflower
Key issue: Motivation
Recommended source: Gaia Essences

Athena – The Warrior
Flower essences: Cyclamen, Fuchsia, Geranium, Verbena
Key issue: Strength
Recommended source: Gaia Essences

Hathor – The Flame
Flower essences: African Violet, Purple Crocus, Purple Iris
Key issue: Inspiration
Recommended source: Gaia Essences

Demeter – Hope
Flower essences: Hellebore, Ivy, Tobacco plant, Thyme, Snowdrop
Key issue: Nurturing
Recommended source: Gaia Essences

Mary – Purification
Flower essences: Gardenia, White Jasmine, Yarrow (white)
Key issue: Truth
Recommended source: Gaia Essences

Samhain Goddess
Flower essences: Mandrake, Mexican Tarragon, Spindle
Key issue: Healing
Recommended source: Sovereignty Essences

Imbolc Goddess
Flower essences: Hazel, Mandrake, Oriental Hellebore, Wallflower
Key issue: Focus
Recommended source: Sovereignty Essences

Lammas Goddess
Flower essences: Rose, St John's Wort, Wormwood
Key issue: Birth, creativity
Recommended source: Sovereignty Essences

Beltane Goddess
Flower essences: Forget-Me-Not, Mandrake, Plum
Key issues: Love and relationships
Recommended source: Sovereignty Essences

Spring Equinox Goddess
Mandrake, Pipil Tzin-Tzintli
Key issue: Expression
Recommended source: Sovereignty Essences

Autumnal Equinox Goddess
Flower essences: Sun Opener, Toloache, White Petunia, Wormwood
Key issue: Decisions
Recommended source: Sovereignty Essences

Summer Solstice Goddess
Flower names: Geranium
Key issue: Joyfulness
Recommended source: Sovereignty Essences

Winter Solstice Goddess
Flower essences: Heartsease, Holly, Ivy, Mandrake, Viburnum, Yew
Key issue: Values
Recommended source: Sovereignty Essences

Essence Directory

For further information on the essences referred to throughout this book, contact Essence World (see the entry below), or individual essence producers.

Alaskan Essences
www.alaskanessences.com
P.O. Box 1090
Victor, MT 59875
USA
Tel: +1 800-545-9309

The Ananda Apothecary
www.anandaapothecary.com
245 30th Street
Boulder, CO 80305
USA
Tel: +1 888-658-7798

Aus Angels
www.ausangels.com
PO Box 192
Gibsons
BC V0N1V0
Canada
Tel: +1 866-477-779

Australian Bush Flower Essences
www.ausflowers.com.au
45 Booralie Road
Terrey Hills, NSW 2084
Australia
Tel: +61 2 9450 1388

Bach Flower Remedies
from Sun Essences
www.sunessence.co.uk
Well Cottage
7 Church Road
Colby, Norwich NR11 7AB
UK
Tel. +44 (0)1263 732942

Bodylink Essences and Essence World
www.essenceworld.com
94 High Street
Eton, Berkshire SL4 6AF
UK
Tel: +44 (0)1753 863214

Desert Alchemy
www.desert-alchemy.com
PO Box 44189
Tucson, AZ 85733
USA
Tel: +1 800-296-5488

Flower Essence Services
www.fesflowers.com
PO Box 1769
Nevada City, CA 95959
USA
Tel: +1 800-548-0075

Flower Sense
www.flowersense.co.uk
19 London End
Beaconsfield
Bucks HP9 2HN
UK
Tel: +44 (0)1494 671775

Fox Mountain
www.floweressencesoffoxmountain.com
PO Box 381
Worthington
MA 01098-0381
USA
Tel: +1 413 238 4291

Gaia Essences
www.gaiaessences.com
28 Glebelands Road
Tiverton
Devon EX16 4EB
UK
Tel: +44 (0)1884 259130

Green Man Essences
www.greenmanessences.com
PO Box 6, Exminster
Exeter, Devon EX6 8YE
UK
Tel: +44 (0)1392 832005

Ilminster Essences
www.drandrew.co.uk
Yarn Barton
Sea, Ilminster
Somerset TA20 0SB
UK
Tel: +44 (0)1460 57475

Korte Essences
www.kortephi.com
PHI Essences BV
Rijksweg Zuid 1
NL- 5951 AM Belfeld
The Netherlands
Tel: +31 77-4 75 42 52

Living Essences of Australia
www.livingessences.com.au
PO Box 355
Scarborough, WA 6019
Australia
Tel: +61 8 94435600

Master's Flower Essences
www.mastersessences.com
14618 Tyler Foote Road
Nevada City, CA 95959
USA
Tel: +1 800-347-3639

Pacific Essences
www.pacificessences.com
PO Box 8317
Victoria, BC V8W 3R9
Canada
Tel: +1 250-384-5560

Reading List

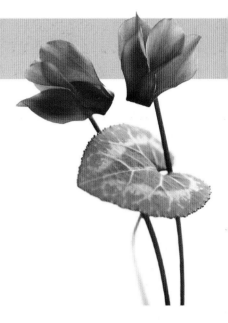

Rainflower Essences
www.rainfloweressence.com
34820 US 19 N
Palm Harbor, FL 34684
USA
Tel: 888-723-7434

Rising Serpent Essences
www.penninehealing.co.uk
21 Barratt Buildings, Burnley Road
Luddendenfoot
Yorkshire HX2 6AA
UK
Tel: +44 (0)1422 882 071

Sabian Essences
www.essenceworld.com
PO Box 527
Kew
Melbourne VIC 3101
Australia
Tel: 161 3 9852 8033

Silvercord Essences
www.silvercord-essences.co.uk
Turnpike Cottage
Chawleigh
Chulmleigh
Devon EX18 7EU
UK
Tel: +44 (0)1769 580 913

Soul Quintessence System
www.soulquintessence.com
6 Millside Court
Church Street
Bookham KT23 3JS
UK
Tel: +44 (0) 1753 863214

The South African Flower Essences
www.safloweressences.co.za
PO Box 721
Constantia, 7847 Cape Town
South Africa
Tel: +27 21 7946762

Sovereignty Essences
Details as for Green Man Essences

Bach, Edward *Heal Thyself: Explanation of the Real Cause and Cure of Disease* CW Daniel Co Ltd, *1996*

Biddulph, Steve *Manhood* Vermilion, 2004

Coelho, Paulo *The Pilgrimage* Harper Collins, 1997

Emery, Kevin Ross *Managing the Gift: Alternative approaches for Attention Deficit Disorder* Lightlines Publishing, 2000

Emoto, Masaru *The Hidden Messages in Water* Pocket Books, 2005

Evans, Patricia *The Verbally Abusive Relationship: How to Recognize it and How to Respond* Adams Media Corporation, 2002

Forward, Susan *Toxic Parents* Bantam Books, 2002

Foundation for Inner Peace *A Course In Miracles* Arkana, 1997

Gerber, Michael *The E Myth Revisted* HarperCollins, 1994

Gerber, Richard *Vibrational Medicine for the 21st Century* Piatkus Books, 2001

Gladwell, Malcolm *Blink: The Power of Thinking Without Thinking* Penguin, 2006

Hay, Louise L *You Can Heal your Life* Hay House, 2002

Jeffers, Susan *Opening Our Hearts to Men* Piatkus, 2005

Judith, Anodea *Wheels of Life: User's Guide to the Chakra System* Llewellyn, 1987

Maltz, Maxwell *Psycho-Cybernetics* Simon & Schuster, 1994

McTaggart, Lynne *The Field: The Quest for the Secret Force of the Universe* HarperCollins, 2003

Millman, Dan *The Life You Were Born to Live* H J Kramer, 1995

Mountain Dreamer, Oriah *The Invitation* HarperCollins, 2000

Myss, Caroline *Anatomy of the Spirit* Bantam, 1997

Norwood, Robin *Women Who Love Too Much* Arrow, 2004

Peck, M Scott *People of the Lie: Hope for Healing Human Evil* Arrow, 1990

Pert, Candace *Molecules of Emotion* Pocket Books, 1999

Redfield, James *The Celestine Prophecy* Bantam, 1994

Ruiz, Don Miguel *The Voice of Knowledge: A Practical Guide to Inner Peace* Amber-Allen Publishing, 2004

Shinn, Florence Scovel *The Game of Life & How to Play it* Vermilion, 2005

Glossary

AURA Force field or energy field around the body. The aura is the combined energy of the body, which emanates from the physical body rather like a cocoon.

CHAKRA Spinning centres within the many layers of the energetic physical body, responsible for relaying messages. First chakra – fear (most complex chakra); second chakra – self-esteem, confidence and creativity; third chakra – ego and drive, willpower, metabolism, assimilation of information, transformation; fourth chakra – love (heart) and breathing, two elements vital for life. All communication lines from other chakras flow through the heart chakra; fifth chakra – communication, in all forms verbal and nonverbal, both internally and externally. Communication with the self and with others, sound, resonance, expression, intonation, physical passion, touch, includes communication from the physical arms and hands; sixth chakra – sight, visualization, vision, inner tuition (intuition); seventh chakra – thoughts and silence (meditation), guidance, information and wisdom, understanding and consciousness.

CROSS ENERGY The energy that originates between the two energetic points, one at each ear, which influence the 'fight or flight' response and operate as part of the body's protective system. The cross energy flows up and down the body – notable power areas are the shoulders, diaphragm, hips, knees, ankles, elbows and wrists. It can increase or decrease in size, vibrancy and protection for the physical body. It supports the aura to help protect the body.
NB When an essence is described as reducing or stopping the cross energy, it is important to remember that essences only work for a particular time, so it will not stop the pulsing indefinitely. You may want to 'take off' the power to help the healing process if you need to slow down or conserve internal energy for internal repair, or to give a much-needed shove to push something out of the thought processes.

EMOTIONAL SUBTLE BODY A parallel body that coexists with the physical body, covering emotions, sensitivities and feelings.

ENERGY MATRIX A circuit around the body, carrying energy and messages between the chakras. There are two – one around the physical body and one around the spiritual body.

KUNDALINI The energy that we connect to through the core of our being, a connection between our navel and our sacral bone. By utilizing it we can plug into our own unique power, or vibration. Each level of vibration has a colour that indicates how high or low it is: if your core colour is red, you work at a lower vibration than someone whose core colour is blue, for instance. Each colour represents your experience as a soul, how you see things and relate to the world. The more spiritual practice you put in, the higher your vibrational colour. When we move from one colour or vibration to another, we automatically go through a period of transition and growth and sometimes experience growing pains in our psyche. Thoughts are challenged and beliefs shift.

MEMBRANE or interface, closely related to the fluids and brain of the dense body. The connection between the physical and spiritual body; the cement that holds us together. It is the first part of our energy field that is affected by trauma and shock and it can hold onto that shock for many years. It is also the storehouse for memories, and plays a vital function in the replay of truth – if we tell fibs or lies to ourselves or others, the normal viscosity of the membrane becomes thicker resulting in a reduced flow-through of energy and ultimately separation.

PHYSICAL BODY The sum of the many layers of energy that encompass the physical body, from the densest of energy, the manifestation of the body on earth, to the very fine layer sitting alongside the membrane.

PHYSICAL VALVE A one-way valve situated at mid-point on the body between the thighs, halfway between the knees and bottom. It works in tandem with inspiration. Debris can get caught up in this one-way system and it sometimes needs flushing out.

SPIRITUAL BODY A parallel body that coexists with the physical body, home of the spirit or soul.

SPIRITUAL VALVE A one-way valve between the heart and the throat slightly higher than the thymus gland, which works in tandem with expiration. Debris can get caught up in this one-way system and it sometimes needs flushing out.

SUBTLE ETHERIC LAYERS/LEVELS Layers or levels that make up the vibrational energy system, or life force.

VAGUS NERVE The tenth cranial nerve, which originates in the brainstem and extends down to the abdomen. It supplies motor fibres to all the organs except the suprarenal glands and is responsible for many tasks, including heart rate, peristalsis-movement in the gut and gag reflex.

The Flower Healer is about the fascinating world of energy and essences and those most selected by people just like you over the past four years using Intuits™. These are not the essences I selected for my patients, but the essences that these people chose for themselves using this system. Originally this process was done manually but for the past three years we have flown into the 21st century and now have a fabulous programme that does the work for us. With our ever increasing sophisticated communication avenues we can even access this from our phones!

By stating their intention, asking a carefully worded question and then choosing a series of numbers, they came up with their own blend of essences. It's as simple as that. Those numbers are utilized to select a quantity of essences, usually four. Intuits™ then produces a recommended blend, unique to your circumstances. After that, the blend is prepared and you then take over the healing process along with your essences.

Intuits™ is a programme developed by me and my intuition. It helps everyone to choose intuitively what they need without their emotions getting in the way. As there are no words used in the selection process there are no emotional associations. It takes the guesswork out of choosing the right essence and lets your body talk to you in ways I never thought possible. The results of this astound me every time it is used.

The research into the outcome of these results is fascinating. Some essences are constantly chosen in one day. A suggestion that it is 'something in the air,' or that the planetary movements are affecting us all, can be accepted. When we see this pattern emerging, we, the staff at Essence World, also take the essence.

We see a trend in geographical areas, too, as our clients can phone for an Intuits™ consultation and are therefore not limited to a personal visit. Seasonal factors and occupations also play their part in the results as do the changes in cats and dogs, which are obvious to the eye but their energy makeup is not. Even the very minute differences between male and female clients become evident!

The implications for this are immense. We get referrals from doctors and vets who 'don't do emotional problems'. This system gives you back your empowerment. You instinctively know what you need, and this system just helps you to access this. Even I use it.

Now due to its phenomenal success, I am training Intuits™ practitioners as the demand dictates that you want to be able to go local and not wait for the post. We already have a practitioner in Australia and have more undergoing training this year from different Australian states. If you would like to know any more about Intuits™ there is information on the website, www.essenceworld.com.

Index

Acknowledgements

A web of many thin threads has come together to produce this book. When I look back to spotlight those that have stood out it seems like a virtually impossible task. If it were not for everything and everyone I have met in my life I wouldn't be me. My teachers are countless and include those in spirit alongside the humans. My patients and clients who put their trust in me, I am truly humbled by their responses and growth in themselves.

But this work would not have been possible without my writing mentor and great friend Jo Glanville-Blackburn. I want to thank Jo for her belief in me and staying up all night by my side tweaking, prodding, laughing and crying when the deadlines were imminent. Jo, what a journey for both of us! To Cindy and Liz from CICO for their insight and encouragement. My beautiful boys, Stuart and Nick, for being my biggest teachers. These guys show more wisdom than their years and bring me back to earth to deal with life when I float off. A big thank you also goes to Tom for taking me out of the dark ages by programming Intuits™. Without this there would be no instant reports and useable information. And last but not least John and Harmony for showing me the way around the world of energy and for taking me by the hand and leading me step by step through the maze of magic.

Picture Credits

AGStockUSA, Inc./Alamy: 85 (bottom right). Miroslava Arnaudova/Flowerphotos: 54 (bottom right), 85 (top right). Arco Images/Alamy: 58 (left), 77 (top left). Ashton/Flowerphotos: 6, 39 (left). Australian National Botanic Gardens: 66 (left), 67 (left & top right), 69 (left & top right), 71 (top right), 72 (left & bottom right), 73 (left), 74 (top right), 78 (left), 86 (top right). Pallava Bagla/Science Picture Library: 50 (right). Lisa Barber/Flowerphotos: 7. John Beedle/Flowerphotos: 42 (left). Niall Benvie/Flowerphotos: 25, 40 (left). Blickwinkel/Alamy: 49 (left), 53 (top right), 68 (bottom right), 80 (top right), 84 (left). Jonathan Buckley/Flowerphotos: 10, 47 (left & top right), 65 (top left). Captureworx/ Flowerphotos: 9. Grace Carlton/Flowerphotos: 47 (bottom right). Roy P. Chatfield/Flowerphotos: 39 (top right), 49 (right), 64 (right). Chinju@digipix/Alamy: 65 (bottom left). Simon Colmer & Abby Rex/Alamy: 81 (right). Geoff Dann: 58 (top right), 76 (left). Danita Delimont/Alamy: 63 (right), 75 (bottom left). Lise Dumont/Alamy: 73 (top right). Dana Edmunds/Alamy: 86 (left). F1 online/Alamy: 74 (bottom right). The Forestry Commission: 44 (right), 48 (left), 51 (bottom right), 53 (left), 56 (left & top right), 59 (top right), 60 (right), 78 (right), 87 (left). Steve Gosling/Flowerphotos: 48 (top right). Graphic Science/Alamy: 30, 51 (top right), 88. Sarah Heneghan/Flowerphotos: 36. Mike Hill/Flowerphotos: 40 (bottom right). Holt Studios International Ltd/Alamy: 53 (bottom). Tony Howell/Flowerphotos: 12. Eric Hunt: 61 (bottom left). Eddie Judd/Flowerphotos: 20. Sue Kennedy/Flowerphotos: 57 (left). Cezary Kuligowski: 75 (right), 77 (bottom right). Alexander Kurlovich/Flowerphotos: 1, 22, 70 (top left). Sue & Simon Lily: 44 (left). Rob Matheson/Flowerphotos: 81 (left). Niall McDiarmid/Alamy: 21, 52 (bottom right). Mediacolor/Alamy: 76 (top right). Nic Miller/Flowerphotos: 22, 40 (top right), 71 (bottom right), 97, 138. Maria Mosolova/Flowerphotos: 45 (bottom right). Nature Photographers Ltd/Alamy: 65 (right). Julian Nieman/Flowerphotos: 15, 45 (left), 48 (bottom right), 51 (bottom left), 96, 101. Barbara Olive: 22, 38 (left), 42 (top & bottom right), 43 (top right), 46 (bottom right), 52 (top right), 59 (left), 61 (bottom right), 66 (top & bottom right), 68 (left & top right), 77 (bottom left), 82 (top & bottom right), 84 (top right), 89, 91, 93. Nick Olive: 74 (left). Martin O'Neil/Flowerphotos: 61 (top right). Gill Orsman/Flowerphotos: 63 (top left). Oxford Scientific: 62 (right), 70 (bottom left). Roy Palmer: 72 (top right), 83 (right). Joerg Pein: 38 (bottom right). Michael Peuckert/Flowerphotos: 41 (top left). Gillian Plummer/Flowerphotos: 54 (top right), 80 (bottom right). Sally Reed/Flowerphotos: 22, 25, 46 (left), 71 (left). Kevin Schafer/Alamy: 59 (bottom right). Leonid Serebrennikov/Alamy: 87 (top right). Carol Sharp/Flowerphotos: 14, 17, 24, 28, 34, 35, 38 (top right), 39 (bottom right), 43 (bottom right), 46 (top right), 50 (left), 51 (top left), 55 (bottom right), 56 (bottom right), 57 (top right), 58 (bottom right), 61 (top left), 62 (left), 63 (bottom left), 69 (bottom right), 70 (right), 79 (bottom left & right), 80 (left), 82 (left), 84 (bottom right), 87 (bottom right), 94, 98, 99, 136. Marilyn Shenton/Alamy: 43 (left). Steve Shipman/Flowerphotos: 83 (left). David Smith/Alamy: 86 (bottom right). Duncan Smith/Flowerphotos: 54 (left), 79 (right), 105. Tim Smith/Flowerphotos: 22, 32, 33, 41 (bottom left & right), 45 (top right), 60 (left). Simon Stirrup/Alamy: 35, 55 (top left). Steve Taylor/Alamy: 57 (bottom right). Andrew Tresidder: 55 (top right). Dave Tully/Flowerphotos: 30, 52 (left), 102. Dave Zubraski/Flowerphotos: 64 (left), 67 (bottom right), 73 (bottom right), 85 (left), 91.